Recent Advances in Coatings of Implant and Dental Biomaterials

Recent Advances in Coatings of Implant and Dental Biomaterials

Editor

Jun-Beom Park

MDPI • Basel • Beijing • Wuhan • Barcelona • Belgrade • Manchester • Tokyo • Cluj • Tianjin

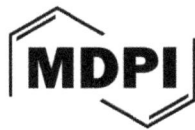

Editor
Jun-Beom Park
The Catholic University of Korea
Korea

Editorial Office
MDPI
St. Alban-Anlage 66
4052 Basel, Switzerland

This is a reprint of articles from the Special Issue published online in the open access journal *Coatings* (ISSN 2079-6412) (available at: https://www.mdpi.com/journal/coatings/special_issues/Recent_Adv_Coat_Implant_Dent_Biomater).

For citation purposes, cite each article independently as indicated on the article page online and as indicated below:

LastName, A.A.; LastName, B.B.; LastName, C.C. Article Title. *Journal Name* **Year**, *Volume Number*, Page Range.

ISBN 978-3-0365-5833-2 (Hbk)
ISBN 978-3-0365-5834-9 (PDF)

© 2022 by the authors. Articles in this book are Open Access and distributed under the Creative Commons Attribution (CC BY) license, which allows users to download, copy and build upon published articles, as long as the author and publisher are properly credited, which ensures maximum dissemination and a wider impact of our publications.

The book as a whole is distributed by MDPI under the terms and conditions of the Creative Commons license CC BY-NC-ND.

Contents

Preface to "Recent Advances in Coatings of Implant and Dental Biomaterials" vii

Ji-Youn Kim and Jun-Beom Park
Various Coated Barrier Membranes for Better Guided Bone Regeneration: A Review
Reprinted from: *Coatings* 2022, *12*, 1059, doi:10.3390/coatings12081059 1

Ricard Aceves-Argemí, Elisabet Roca-Millan, Beatriz González-Navarro, Antonio Marí-Roig, Eugenio Velasco-Ortega and José López-López
Titanium Meshes in Guided Bone Regeneration: A Systematic Review
Reprinted from: *Coatings* 2021, *11*, 316, doi:10.3390/coatings11030316 15

Jing Chen, Wenxiu Que, Bo Lei and Beibei Li
Highly Bioactive Elastomeric Hybrid Nanoceramics for Guiding Bone Tissue Regeneration
Reprinted from: *Coatings* 2022, *12*, 1633, doi:10.3390/coatings12111633 29

Santiago Arango-Santander, Lina Serna, Juliana Sanchez-Garzon and John Franco
Evaluation of *Streptococcus mutans* Adhesion to Stainless Steel Surfaces Modified Using Different Topographies Following a Biomimetic Approach
Reprinted from: *Coatings* 2021, *11*, 829, doi:10.3390/coatings11070829 41

Chang-Joo Park, Jae Hyung Lim, Marco Tallarico, Kyung-Gyun Hwang, Hyook Choi, Gyu-Jang Cho, Chang Kim, Il-Seok Jang, Ju-Dong Song, Amy M. Kwon, Sang Ho Jeon and Hyun-Kyung Park
Coating of a Sand-Blasted and Acid-Etched Implant Surface with a pH-Buffering Agent after Vacuum-UV Photofunctionalization
Reprinted from: *Coatings* 2020, *10*, 1040, doi:10.3390/coatings10111040 53

Wilhelmus F. Bouwman, Nathalie Bravenboer, Christiaan M. ten Bruggenkate and Engelbert A.J. M. Schulten
The Use of Autogenous Bone Mixed with a Biphasic Calcium Phosphate in a Maxillary Sinus Floor Elevation Procedure with a 6-Month Healing Time: A Clinical, Radiological, Histological and Histomorphometric Evaluation
Reprinted from: *Coatings* 2020, *10*, 462, doi:10.3390/coatings10050462 65

Jae-Yong Tae, Yoon-Hee Park, Youngkyung Ko and Jun-Beom Park
The Effects of Bone Morphogenetic Protein-4 on Cellular Viability, Osteogenic Potential, and Global Gene Expression on Gingiva-Derived Stem Cell Spheroids
Reprinted from: *Coatings* 2020, *10*, 1055, doi:10.3390/coatings10111055 79

Jia He, Xiaofeng Yang, Fan Liu, Duo Li, Bowen Zheng, Adil Othman Abdullah and Yi Liu
The Impact of Curcumin on Bone Osteogenic Promotion of MC3T3 Cells under High Glucose Conditions and Enhanced Bone Formation in Diabetic Mice
Reprinted from: *Coatings* 2020, *10*, 258, doi:10.3390/coatings10030258 95

Donghee Lee, Jun-Beom Park, Dani Song, Hye-Min Kim and Sin-Young Kim
Cytotoxicity and Mineralization Potential of Four Calcium Silicate-Based Cements on Human Gingiva-Derived Stem Cells
Reprinted from: *Coatings* 2020, *10*, 279, doi:10.3390/coatings10030279 107

Aina Torrejon-Moya, Alina Apalimova, Beatriz González-Navarro, Ramiro Zaera-Le Gal, Antonio Marí-Roig and José López-López
Calcium Sulfate in Implantology (Biphasic Calcium Sul-Fate/Hydroxyapatite, BCS/HA, Bond Apatite®): Review of the Literature and Case Reports
Reprinted from: *Coatings* **2022**, *12*, 1350, doi:10.3390/coatings12091350 . . . . **119**

Preface to "Recent Advances in Coatings of Implant and Dental Biomaterials"

Recently, the development of coatings of implant and bone surfaces has received a significant amount of interest. The coating of implants may enhance osseointegration. Moreover, coating the surface of implants may provide antimicrobial effects. Various methods/techniques can be applied for coating dental/implant surfaces. Plasma splaying and electrospraying have been developed as coating methods, and a variety of materials have been applied for surface coatings. Growth factors have been used, along with bioactive glasses and ceramics. Similarly, bone surfaces have been coated using various methods to enhance the functionality of the graft material.

Jun-Beom Park
Editor

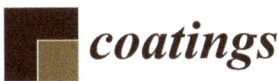

Review

Various Coated Barrier Membranes for Better Guided Bone Regeneration: A Review

Ji-Youn Kim [1] and Jun-Beom Park [2],*

[1] Division of Oral and Maxillofacial Surgery, Department of Dentistry, College of Medicine, St. Vincent's Hospital, The Catholic University of Korea, Seoul 06591, Korea; kimjy@catholic.ac.kr
[2] Department of Periodontics, College of Medicine, The Catholic University of Korea, Seoul 06591, Korea
* Correspondence: jbassoon@catholic.ac.kr; Tel.: +82-22258-6290

Abstract: A good barrier membrane is one of the important factors for effective guided bone/tissue regeneration (GBR/GTR) in the case of periodontal bone defects. Several methods are being discussed to overcome and improve the shortcomings of commercially available membranes. One of the methods is to coat the membrane with bioactive materials. In this study, 41 studies related to coated membranes for GBR/GTR published in the last 5 years were reviewed. These studies reported coating the membrane with various bioactive materials through different techniques to improve osteogenesis, antimicrobial properties, and physical/mechanical properties. The reported studies have been classified and discussed based on the purpose of coating. The goal of the most actively studied research on coating or surface modification of membranes is to improve new bone formation. For this purpose, calcium phosphate, bioactive glass, polydopamine, osteoinduced drugs, chitosan, platelet-rich fibrin, enamel matrix derivatives, amelotin, hyaluronic acid, tantalum, and copper were used as membrane coating materials. The paradigm of barrier membranes is changing from only inert (or biocompatible) physical barriers to bioactive osteo-immunomodulatory for effective guided bone and tissue regeneration. However, there is a limitation that there exists only a few clinical studies on humans to date. Efforts are needed to implement the use of coated membranes from the laboratory bench to the dental chair unit. Further clinical studies are needed in the patients' group for long-term follow-up to confirm the effect of various coating materials.

Keywords: anti-bacterial agents; calcium phosphate; guided tissue regeneration; membranes; osteogenesis

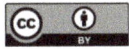

1. Introduction

Many elderly patients with bone loss and tooth loss owed to periodontal disease visit the dentist in an aging society [1]. Sufficient alveolar bone regeneration is essential for successful periodontal treatment or dental implant treatment. However, compared to soft tissue, bone has a relatively low regeneration potential [2]. In guided bone regeneration (GBR) or guided tissue regeneration (GTR) treatment, factors such as barrier membranes, the skillful technique of dentists, healthy patients, and bone materials play an important role. Among them, the membrane used for GTR/GBR prevents invasion of the soft tissue into bone defects due to the fast growth rate of fibroblasts outwards and serves to maintain appropriate space inwards, thereby allowing sufficient time for bone regeneration [2,3]. Therefore, the membrane should have characteristics such as (1) biocompatibility to prevent soft tissue dehiscence and minimize tissue reactions, (2) space maintenance and structural integrity, (3) host tissue integration, and (4) an ease of handling during surgery with no memory [4].

The commercially available membranes that are currently used can be broadly divided into two types: non-resorbable membranes and resorbable membranes. Representative examples of non-resorbable membranes include expanded polytetrafluoroethylene (ePTFE)

and titanium (Ti) mesh. Their advantage is that they have the properties of good intensity and barrier effects. Especially, the Ti membrane could be deformed to suit various forms of bone defect and maintain the extensive space because of their high rigidity and plasticity [5]. However, the disadvantages include poor cellular adhesion, slower cellular growth, bone regeneration, and the need for secondary surgery, which may lead to secondary trauma to the gum [6,7]. Besides, the exposed non-resorbable membranes easily form a biofilm in the oral cavity and may experience failure of bone regeneration due to bacterial infection [8,9]. On the contrary, the resorbable membrane has a great advantage as it does not require secondary surgery for the removal after the regeneration of alveolar bone. In addition, it has advantages such as good biocompatibility, weak immunogenicity, higher cell adhesion, and tissue healing properties [10]. Representative resorbable membranes include collagen membranes made from a bovine or porcine source and biodegradable synthetic polymer membranes [11]. However, collagen membrane has disadvantages such as insufficient mechanical properties and a fast degradation speed that is short to maintain sufficient space for an appropriate time as a barrier [10]. Biodegradable polymer membranes, such as poly(L-lactide) (PLLA), has advanced mechanical properties but are associated with inherent shortcomings such as hydrophobicity, poor cellular affinity, and osteoconductive activity compared to collagen membrane [12].

Therefore, to compensate for these shortcomings and increase bone regeneration, research on the development of coating or the surface treatment of membranes have been conducted continuously. The technology of coating continues to develop, especially in membrane application. Coating of the membrane with various materials can be applied for GTR applications as bioactive and anti-bacterial purposes [13]. However, there exists only a few review papers focusing on the coating or surface treatment of barrier membranes. In this study, we have reviewed barrier membrane coating-related papers published in the last 5 years, investigated the research conducted to date, and seek the direction of development of coated membranes in the future.

2. Materials and Methods

A literature search was performed in electronic databases, including PubMed, Medline, OVID, and Web of Science, by using the following keywords: "membranes", "guided bone regeneration", "guided tissue regeneration", "coated", and "coating" from 2017 January to 2022 June. Documents written in English were selected. Sixty-two papers were found and among them, a total of 41 papers were included in this study, excluding 21 papers not related to coated membranes or review papers (Figure 1). Based on the selected 41 papers, we would like to briefly review the membrane coating materials studied so far (Table 1).

Table 1. Summary of included studies on coated barrier membranes.

Improved Property	Coated Materials	Resorbable Membrane					Non-Resorbable Membrane	
		Collagen	Synthetic Polymer	SA, Chitosan	Mg Mesh	Ti Mesh	PTFE, PP, Nylon	
Osteogenesis	CaP, HA, TCP	Chu et al. [14], Dau et al. [15], Dubus et al. [16], Yang et al. [17]	Higuchi et al. [18], Van et al. [19], Torres-Lagares et al. [20], Torres-Lagares et al. [21]	-	Byun et al. [22]	Nguyen et al. [23]	-	
	Bioactive glass, SiO$_2$	Chen et al. [2], Dau et al. [15]	Shi et al. [24], Torres-Lagares et al. [21], Terzopoulou et al. [25], Lian et al. [26], Castillo-Dalí et al. [27]	-	-	-	-	
	Polydopamine	-	Chen et al. [12], Lee et al. [28], Hasani-Sadrabadi et al. [29], Wang et al. [30], Shi et al. [24], Liu et al. [31]	Xu et al. [32]	-	-	Ejeian et al. [33]	

Table 1. Cont.

Improved Property	Coated Materials	Resorbable Membrane			Non-Resorbable Membrane		
		Collagen	Synthetic Polymer	SA, Chitosan	Mg Mesh	Ti Mesh	PTFE, PP, Nylon
	Drugs	van Oirschot et al. [34], van de Ven et al. [35]	Terzopoulou et al. [25], Lian et al. [26]	-	-	-	-
	Chitosan	Dubus et al. [16],	Porrelli et al. [36]	-	Guo et al. [37]	-	-
	PRF, EMD, AMTN	Kapa et al. [38], Miron et al. [9], Ikeda et al. [39]	Ikeda et al. [39]	-	-	-	-
	HyA	Dubus et al. [16], Silva et al. [40]	Van et al. [19]	-	-	-	-
	Tantalum	-	Hwang et al. [41]	-	-	-	-
	Lactoferrin	-	Lee et al. [28]	-	-	-	-
	Cuprous oxide	-	-	Xu et al. [32]	-	-	-
	Strontium	Yang et al. [17]	-	-	-	Nguyen et al. [23]	-
Antimicrobial property	Silver nanoparticles	Chen et al. [42]	Porrelli et al. [36], Wang et al. [30]	-	-	-	-
	Antibiotic drugs	-	Shi et al. [24], Lian et al. [26]	-	-	Zhao et al. [43]	-
	CHX, AMPs	-	-	Boda et al. [44]	-	-	-
	Cuprous oxide	-	-	Xu et al. [32]	-	-	-
	FN-silk, pectin	-	-	Boda et al. [44]	-	-	Tasiopoulos et al. [45]
	Ti, Mg	Choy et al. [46]	Zhang et al. [47]	-	-	-	-
Physical/mechanical property	Graphene oxide	De Marco et al. [48]	-	-	-	-	-
	EGCG	Chu et al. [14]	-	-	-	-	-
	Chitosan	-	-	-	Guo et al. [37]	Zhao et al. [43]	Fernandes et al. [49]
	Polydopamine	-	Chen et al. [12]	-	-	-	-
	AMTN	Ikeda et al. [39]	Ikeda et al. [39]	-	-	-	-
	HA	-	-	-	Byun et al. [22]	-	-
No significant difference	II and PVD (Mg)	-	-	-	Steigmann et al. [50]	-	-
	APP (Ti)	-	-	-	Toyama et al. [51]	-	-

Abbreviation: SA, sodium alginate hydrogel composite; Mg, magnesium; Ti, titanium; PTFE, polytetrafluoroethylene; PP, polypropylene; CaP, calcium phosphate; HA, hydroxyapatite; TCP, β-tricalcium phosphate; SiO_2, silicon dioxide; PRF, platelet-rich fibrin; EMD, enamel matrix derivative; AMTN, amelotin; HyA, hyaluronic acid; CHX, chlorhexidine; AMPs, antimicrobial peptides; FN-silk, recombinant spider silk protein functionalized with a cell-binding motif from fibronectin; EGCG, epigallocatechin-3-gallate; II, ion implantation; PVD, physical vaper deposition; APP, atmospheric pressure plasma treatment.

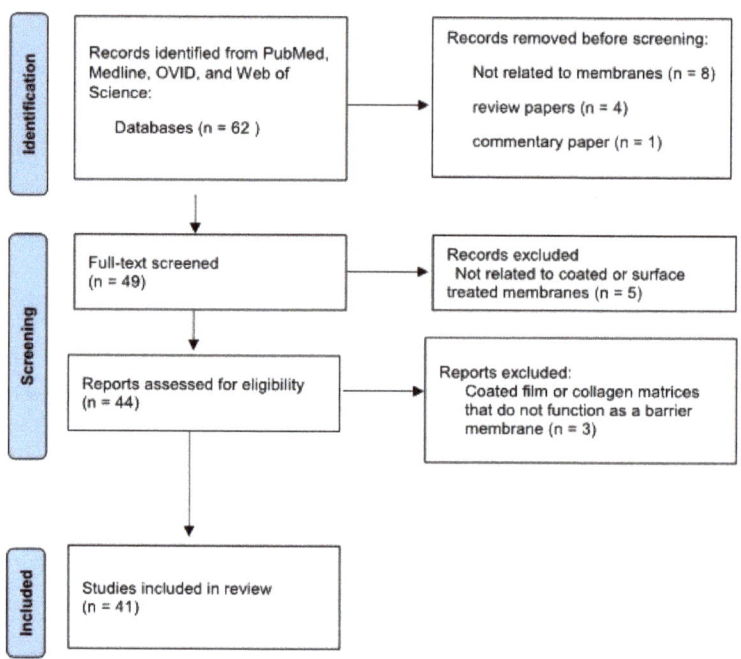

Figure 1. This is the flow chart of this study.

3. Results

3.1. Improved Osteogenesis

Various interdisciplinary approaches of surface coating have been performed in terms of biomaterials, drug release, and therapeutic effects [52]. The goal of the most actively studied research on coating or the surface modification of membranes is to improve new bone formation. For this purpose, calcium phosphate (CaP), bioactive glass, polydopamine (PDA), osteoinduced drugs, chitosan, platelet-rich fibrin (PRF), enamel matrix derivatives (EMT), amelotin (AMTN), hyaluronic acid (HyA), tantalum (Ta), and copper were used as membrane coating materials.

3.1.1. Calcium Phosphate, Hydroxyapatite, and β-Tricalcium Phosphate

CaP belongs to the family of minerals containing calcium cations (Ca^{2+}) together with inorganic phosphate anions, which are abundant in native human bone and teeth [53]. CaP is a representative bioactive material [53]. The calcium ion induces the proliferation and differentiation of human mesenchymal stem cells (MSCs), stimulates osteoblastic bone synthesis by activating the extracellular signal-regulated kinase 1/2 pathway and phosphatidylinositol 3-kinase/Akt pathways [53–56]. In addition, phosphate regulates the proliferation and differentiation of the osteoblasts and increases the expression of BMPs [53,57,58]. CaP demonstrates osteoconductivity and osteoinductivity characteristics through the above cell signaling pathways as well as good biocompatibility, non-immunogenicity, and non-inflammatory behavior [59]. CaP has been utilized to improve bone regeneration in ways such as increasing osteoconductivity for bone ingrowth, enhancing osteoinductivity for bone mineralization with ion release control, and encapsulating drugs or growth factors [59,60]. Hydroxyapatite (HA, ($Ca_5(PO_4)_3(OH)$)) and β-tricalcium phosphate (TCP, ($Ca_3(PO_4)_2$)) are also included in this family [53]. HA constitutes the largest amount of inorganic components in human bone [61]. Calcium phosphate has been studied for bone regenerative treatment as a coating material for membrane and dental implants, and also as a raw material [53].

In 2017, Chu et al. studied nanostructured HA (nanoHA)-coated epigallocatechin-3-gallate (EGCG) cross-linked collagen membranes [14]. In this in vivo study, nanoHA-coated and EGCG cross-linked collagen membranes showed the highest bone healing efficacy [14]. Furthermore, due to EGCG, the membrane showed improved mechanical properties, such as elasticity and thermal stability [14]. In 2019, Nguyen et al. studied strontium (Sr)-doped CaP-coated Ti mesh membranes. Both Sr- and CaP-coated Ti mesh presented the highest percentages of bone–mesh contact in the critical bone defect animal model [23]. In 2019, Higuchi et al. used electrospraying or sonocoating methods for nanoHA coating of Poly(D,L-lactic acid), (PDLLA)/Poly(D,L-lactide-co-glycolide) (PLGA) membranes. In this study, nanoHA sonocoated polymer membranes showed better cellular metabolic activity than non-coated control membranes [18].

3.1.2. Bioactive Glass and Silicon Dioxide

The form and application of glass have developed along with the development of human civilization for thousands of years [62]. Since the late 1960s, various combinations of bioactive glasses for regenerative medicine have been developed and improved [62]. Due to the bonding ability of bioactive glasses to both hard and soft tissues, and osteoconductive, osteoinductive, and angiogenesis properties, the material is considered a third-generation biomedical material [62–65]. Numerous pieces of research on the bioactive glass coating on dental implants and membranes are ongoing to enhance bone regeneration and induce fast tissue bonding [2,27,66,67]. Furthermore, for improved physical, functional, and chemical properties, the bioactive glasses are incorporated with different ions (e.g., Sr, Cu, Zn, etc.), osteo-induced drugs (bisphosphonate and dexamethasone), and nanoHA [2,15,21,25,26,68].

In 2018, Chen et al. reported a nanometer-sized bioactive glass $Ca_2ZnSi_2O_7$-coated collagen membrane via a pulsed laser deposition coating technique [2]. This study showed that the expression of osteogenic factors was upregulated and osteogenic differentiation of bone marrow stem cells was enhanced in the coated membrane group, attributable to coated nutrient bioactive glass [2]. In 2020, Dau et al. reported SiO_2-enhanced nanoHA-coated collagen membranes via the spin–spray coating method [15]. In this study, SiO_2-enhanced nanoHA-coated collagen membranes showed the fastest and most pronounced vascularization properties [15]. In 2019, Terzopoulou et al. reported ibandronate-loaded bioactive glasses-coated poly(ε-caprolactone) (PCL) membrane [25]. In the reported study, two different synthesized mesoporous bioactive glasses (SiO_2-CaO-P_2O_5 and SiO_2-SrO-P_2O_5) were loaded with ibandronate and coated on PCL membranes by the spin coating technique. Both the bioactive glasses demonstrated an increase in hydrophilicity and bioactivity, especially in the ibandronate-loaded and Sr-substituted bioactive glass-coated membranes [25].

3.1.3. Polydopamine and Polydopamine Platform with Other Substances

PDA has been known as one of the most efficient universal surface-coating materials due to its ability to strongly attach to almost all kinds of substrates, since its first report in 2007 [69,70]. PDA has been reported to promote cellular adhesion and mineral deposition of hydroxyapatite [29,71,72]. In addition, PDA is a good platform for surface tethering and releasing small molecules for tailoring the functionality of PDA. The target molecules (polymers, proteins, peptides, and drugs) could be readily immobilized on PDA by ad-layer formation or one-pot coating technique [73–75].

In 2019, Hasani-Sadrabadi et al. developed biomimetic PDA-coated PCL membranes via the membrane immersion technique using dopamine hydrochloride to promote adhesion [29]. In this study, the coated PDA layer was identified to accelerate the osteogenic differentiation of MSCs by promoting hydroxyapatite mineralization [29]. In 2019, Chen et al. reported that the PDA-coated PLLA membrane improved hydrophilicity, cytocompatibility, tensile properties, and osteogenic activity [12], and the membrane was soaked in

1.5 times stimulated body fluid for the biomineralization of HA. In this in vitro study, HA immobilization and PDA coating played a synergistic osteoconductive effect [12]. In 2020, Ejeian et al. reported in situ crystallization of zeolitic imidazolate framework-8 (ZIF-8) on the PDA-modified polypropylene (PP) membrane [33]. The ZIF-8/PDA/PP membrane showed significantly increased osteogenic differentiation of dental pulp stem cells, as well as increased physical properties. In 2022, Lee et al. reported that lactoferrin immobilized the PLLA/PCL membrane by using the polydopamine coating technique [28]. Lactoferrin is known to exhibit biological functional activities such as bone regeneration and anti-inflammation [28,76,77]. In this study, the lactoferrin–polydopamine-coated PLLA/PCL membrane showed enhanced osteoinductive and anti-inflammatory activities compared to only the PDL-coated membrane [28].

3.1.4. Drugs for Osteogenesis: Bisphosphonate with or without Testosterone and Dexamethasone

As anti-osteoporotic drugs, the bisphosphonates (e.g., alendronate, ibandronate, and zoledronate, etc.) interfere with the bone turnover process through inactivation of the osteoclast activity, thereby resulting in reduced bone breakdown [1,34]. The bisphosphonates prevent osteoporotic pathologic fractures and improved bone regeneration [34,78]. However, it could also be a causative agent for medication-related osteonecrosis of the jaw [1]. Testosterone is another important osteoanabolic agent in men, that stimulates the proliferation of preosteoblasts and the differentiation of osteoblasts [79]. Currently, bisphosphonate and testosterone combination therapy has been exploited for the synergistic stimulation of bone regeneration [34,35]. As a synthetic glucocorticoid, locally delivered dexamethasone (Dex) showed great osteogenic induction of MSCs [76]. However, the inappropriate systemic delivery of glucocorticoids may cause side effects such as hyperglycemia, immunosuppression, and osteoporosis [76,80].

In 2020, van Oirschot et al., and in 2021, van den Ven et al., reported a testosterone and alendronate ultrasonic spray-coated collagen membrane by using PLGA 5004A as a carrier [34,35]. The drug-coated membranes showed superior bone regeneration to the control group with 124% in the minipig bone defect model and 160% in the rat critical-size calvarial defect model [34,35]. In 2019, Lian et al. reported dexamethasone-loaded mesoporous silica nanoparticle-coated PLGA and gelatin composite membranes [26]. In this in vitro experiment, the coated membrane showed an enhanced osteoinductive capacity for rat bone marrow stem cells (BMSCs).

3.1.5. Chitosan

Chitosan derived from the deacetylation of chitin derivatives is one of the most important natural polymers and has been reported to induce osteogenesis and enhanced tissue healing [11,81]. It has biocompatible, self-resorbable, antimicrobial, and economical properties [11]. Though it has poor mechanical properties and a low degradation rate, chitosan plays a role in improving the biological, physical, mechanical, and antimicrobial properties of the membranes either alone or in combination with other functional coating materials [36,37,43,49]. Guo et al. reported a chitosan-coated magnesium (Mg) membrane [37]. In this study, chitosan was used to reduce the degradation rate of the Mg membrane and enhance osteogenic activity. The results showed that the chitosan-coated Mg membrane had a suitable degradation rate and a higher osteogenic potential [37]. However, mechanical properties may not be maintained once degradation begins. In 2021, Porrelli et al. reported that silver nanoparticles (nAgs) stabilized a bioactive lactose-modified chitosan-coated PCL membrane [36]. The nAgs lactose-modified chitosan-coated membrane showed enhanced hydrophilic properties, improved osteoblastic adhesion, proliferation, and discouraged biofilm formation without cytotoxicity [36].

3.1.6. Platelet-Rich Fibrin, Enamel Matrix Derivatives, and Amelotin

PRF, as one of the forms of platelet concentrates, is obtained from the autologous venous blood in the glass-coated tube after centrifugation at 400 g. The PRF contains platelets and their byproducts released during platelet activation. These include numerous growth factors, circulating cytokines, glycoproteins, and fibrin-associated glycan chains that are crucial factors for tissue regeneration [82]. In 2020, Kapa et al. reported the clinical study about the treatment with PRF-coated bones and PRF-coated collagen membranes in sixteen patients with gingival recession due to the loss of alveolar bone and soft gingival tissue [38]. In the study, twelve out of the sixteen patients achieved complete healing of gingival recession, and an increase in gingival thickness was observed in all patients [38].

Like PRF, the extract of porcine embryonic enamel matrix termed 'EMD' has been reported to induce mesenchymal cells to mimic the processes of the development of the tooth and has been broadly used for periodontal regenerative treatment [83]. In 2017, Miron et al. reported the EMD in a liquid carrier system coated with a collagen membrane [9]. The EMD-coated collagen membrane showed increased cell adhesion, osteodifferentiation, and mineralization in an in vitro study.

AMTN, an enamel protein expressed by ameloblasts, is known to play an important role in enamel mineralization [84,85]. Furthermore, the AMTN is known to promote HA mineralization [86]. In 2022, Ikeda et al. reported a collagen hydrogel incorporated with rhAMTN (rhAMTN gel)-coated collagen or polyglactin-woven mesh membranes [39]. The AMTN gel-coated membranes showed accelerated mineralization and adhesion.

3.1.7. Hyaluronic Acid

HyA, a natural linear glycosaminoglycan, is one of the components of the extracellular matrix, and its presence has been documented in skin, aorta, cartilage, and brain [87]. The HyA has hygroscopic, viscoelastic, biocompatible, biodegradable, anti-inflammatory, and bacteriostatic properties [88,89]. Furthermore, it has been reported to induce and enhance cell proliferation, migration, adhesion, and angiogenesis [90,91]. For its ideal regeneration properties, HyA has been widely used in the medical field for orthopedic surgery in the form of intraarticular injection into the osteoarthritic joint and in plastic surgery for dermal regeneration and soft tissue augmentation [87]. In dentistry, HyA has been applied for the treatment of osteoarthritic temporomandibular joint disease and periodontitis [40,92,93].

In 2017, Silva et al. reported that a HyA-coated collagen membrane by using the soaking coating technique did not show a significant difference in new bone formation compared to the non-coated collagen membrane group in rats [40]. However, other studies demonstrated that HyA coated with CaP and chitosan into a collagen membrane through a spraying technique or a HyA- and TCP-modified PCL membrane by the spin-coating technique showed significantly different results in in vitro experiments [16,19]. Dubus et al. [16] reported that a HyA-, CaP-, and chitosan-coated collagen membrane enhanced the proliferation of MSCs and the secretion of cytokines and growth factors. However, further in vivo studies are needed to confirm the effective role of HyA in bone regeneration.

3.1.8. Other Coating Materials—Tantalum, Copper

Ta is known to increase osteoconductivity by promoting the formation of CaP surface layers and is also known to have superior biocompatibility and mechanical properties [94–96]. In 2020, Hwang et al. reported a Ta coated-PLA membrane using sputtered Ta ions using a DC magnetron sputterer to enhance the bioactivity of the PLA membrane [41]. In the reported study, the Ta-coated PLA membrane showed more advanced osteoconductivity than the uncoated PLA membrane in both in vitro and in vivo experiments.

Copper has been known to have attractive dual functions in regenerative medicine [32,97]. Cuprous oxide (CuO_2) nanoparticles have a high efficiency and broad-spectrum antibacterial properties [98]. In addition, Cu^{2+} has been reported to induce the osteogenic differentiation of BMSCs [97]. In 2020, Xu et al. reported a sodium alginate hydrogel composite (CTP-SA) doped with cubic CuO_2 and PDA-coated titanium dioxide (TiO_2) nanoparticles for guided tissue regeneration [32]. In this study, CuO_2 PDA/TiO_2-modified CTP-SA showed improved antibacterial and osteogenic properties according to dual light controls [32].

3.2. Improved Antimicrobial Properties

Besides the previously mentioned CuO_2, nAgs, metronidazole (MNA), doxycycline (Dox), chlorhexidine (CHX), and antimicrobial peptides (AMPs) have been used to improve the antimicrobial properties of the membranes [32].

3.2.1. Silver Nanoparticles

Silver is well known to have broad-spectrum antibacterial properties and has been used in various forms due to its low cytotoxicity [99,100]. Many studies have demonstrated the important activity of Ag nanoparticles (nAgs) against bacterial biofilms [101–104]. There exist studies on the promotion of antimicrobial activity using nAg as a coating material for membranes in the oral cavity [30,36,42]. In 2018, Chen et al. reported nAgs-coated collagen membranes through sonication coating or the sputtering coating technique [42]. The nAgs-coated membranes showed excellent antibacterial effects against *Staphylococcus aureus* and *Pseudomonas aeruginosa*, and exhibited advanced anti-inflammatory effects by reducing the expression and release of inflammatory cytokines [42]. In 2020, Wang et al. reported that nAgs immobilized a PDA-coated PLLA membrane that showed advanced antibacterial effects against *S. aureus* and a good biocompatibility due to low cytotoxicity [30].

3.2.2. Antibiotic Drugs

In 2019, Shi et al. reported an infection-responsive membrane that was esterified MNA-grafted PDA functionalized with a siloxane-coated PCL membrane [24]. The ester bonds could be selectively hydrolyzed by cholesterol esterase (CE) secreted by macrophagocytes accumulated at the site of infection. Thus, the membrane was designed in a manner that increases the CE concentration due to severe infection leading to the release of a higher amount of MNA, thereby resulting in an enhanced antibacterial property. In this study, released MNA due to CE from an MNA-grafted PDA-coated membrane exhibited antibacterial activity [24].

The other studies reported Dox-coated membranes with enhanced antibacterial activities [26,43]. Zhao et al. reported porous chitosan/gelatin/Dox-coated Ti-niobium membrane [43]. Lian et al. reported a Dox-modified PLGA membrane [26].

3.2.3. Chlorhexidine and Antimicrobial Peptides

In 2020, Boda et al. reported an AMPs- or CHX-loaded oxidized pectin-coated chitosan membrane [44]. The D-enantiomer of GL13K (D-GL13K) derived from the human salivary parotid secretory protein and the L-enantiomer of innate defense regulator—1018 (IDR-1018)—were used as AMPs. CHX, D-GL13K, and IDR-1018 were coated on the membrane via the co-electrospinning method or the surface absorption method. In this study, the AMPs-loaded pectin-coated chitosan membrane showed an antimicrobial property that was comparable to CHX against *Streptococci* [44].

3.3. Improved Physical/Mechanical Properties

In addition to EGCG, chitosan, PDA, and AMTN, various materials have been employed to improve the physical and mechanical properties of the membrane [12,14,37,39,43,49].

3.3.1. Recombinant Spider Silk Proteins and Pectin Derivatives for Improved Cell Adhesion

Natural silk has been applied for dental fields due to the structure and features that make it biocompatible [105]. Synthetic polymer membranes are inert and biocompatible; however, they are hydrophobic and less prone to cellular adhesive physical properties [6]. Recombinant spider silk protein not only demonstrates great mechanical characteristics such as strength and elasticity but also great biological characteristics such as biocompatibility, biodegradability, and improved wetting capacity [106,107]. In 2020, Tasiopoulos et al. reported recombinant spider silk protein with a cell-binding motif from a fibronectin (FN-silk)-coated PTFE membrane [45]. In this study, the FN-silk-coated membrane showed higher cell adherence and proliferation properties in both human keratinocytes from soft tissue and human osteosarcoma cells from bone [45].

Pectin is structurally and functionally the most complex polysaccharide present in plant cell walls [108]. Pectin plays important roles in not only mediating plant growth, morphology, and development, but also in gelling and stabilizing the polymers in various foods and medicines [108,109]. Boda et al. reported an oxidized pectin-coated chitosan membrane [44]. The pectin-coated side of the membrane showed a two-fold increase in the mucoadhesive property to the mucosal mimic porcine esophagus than the non-coated side. On the contrary, the non-coated side of the chitosan membrane showed a 3–4 fold stronger adhesion to hard tissue mimicking hydroxyapatite discs than the pectin-coated side [44].

3.3.2. Metal Reinforcement—Titanium and Magnesium

Choy et al. reported a vapor-phase Ti-infiltrated collagen membrane via titanium oxide atomic layer deposition [46]. The Ti-coated collagen membrane led to enhancement in both the tensile strength and Young's modulus compared to the non-coated collagen membrane. Furthermore, the Ti-coated membrane was retained for a longer time than a non-coated collagen membrane that was rapidly degraded by up to 90% within 1 week [46].

Zhang et al. reported a Mg core-reinforced PLA membrane to improve the mechanical–physical properties [47]. The membrane was fabricated by combining two PLA membranes with a fluoride-coated AZ91 (9 wt% Al, 1 wt% Zn) (FAZ91) Mg alloy core by hot pressing. Compared to only the PLA membrane control group, the FAZ91—Mg-reinforced PLA membrane group showed a significantly higher maximum load, stiffness, and faster degradation because FAZ81-Mg promoted the absorption and the degradation of the PLA wrap but was not too delayed [47].

3.3.3. Graphene Oxide

Graphene is a flat monolayer of carbon atoms that are tightly packed into a 2-dimensional honeycomb lattice [110]. Due to its solubility in water and biocompatibility, graphene oxide (GO) has been used as biomaterials [48,111]. De Marco et al. reported a GO-coated collagen membrane [48]. The GO-coated membrane showed a lower deformability with a higher stiffness, an increased roughness, and an increase in the total surface that was exposed to the cells [48].

3.4. No Significant Difference

There exist studies about coated membranes that showed no significant advanced effect compared to the control group.

In 2017, Byun et al. reported a HA-coated Mg membrane to improve biocompatibility [22]. In the result, there were no significant differences or new bone volume, bone volume fraction, or bone surface density between the HA-coated Mg group and the control group [22].

In 2020, Steigmann et al. reported an ion implantation (II) and physical vapor deposition (PVD)-treated Mg membrane to improve biocompatibility [50]. In this study, the PVD-coated membrane demonstrated the absence of a positive influence on the gas cavity formation and advanced immune response compared to the noncoated Mg membrane. The authors concluded that a pure Mg membrane represents a promising alternative to the non-resorbable membrane [50].

In 2020, Toyama et al. reported an atmospheric pressure plasma (APP)-treated Ti membrane and analyzed its effect on the differentiation of BMSCs [51]. In this study, the APP-coated Ti membrane was identified to increase cell migration and gene-level expression of osteogenic markers; however, the suppression of mineralization was observed in an in vitro experiment. Furthermore, in the in vivo experiment, the new bone formation was not significantly different between APP-coated and noncoated Ti membranes [51].

4. Conclusions

The paradigm of the barrier membrane is changing from only inert (or biocompatible) physical barriers to bioactive osteo-immunomodulatory for effective guided bone and tissue regeneration. For this purpose, numerous studies on coating various bioactive materials on the membrane to improve osteogenesis, antimicrobial properties, and physical/mechanical properties by various techniques have been performed. However, there is a limitation that there exists only a few clinical studies on humans to date. Efforts are needed to implement the use of coated membranes from the laboratory bench to the dental chair unit. Further clinical studies are needed in the patients' group for long-term follow-up to confirm the effect of various coating materials.

Author Contributions: Conceptualization, J.-Y.K. and J.-B.P.; methodology, J.-Y.K. and J.-B.P.; formal analysis, J.-Y.K. and J.-B.P.; writing—original draft preparation, J.-Y.K. and J.-B.P.; writing—review and editing. All authors have read and agreed to the published version of the manuscript.

Funding: This research received no external funding.

Institutional Review Board Statement: Not applicable.

Informed Consent Statement: Not applicable.

Data Availability Statement: All data analyzed during this study are included in this published article.

Conflicts of Interest: The authors declare no conflict of interest.

References

1. Kim, J.-Y.; Song, H.C.; Jee, H.-G. Refractory healing after surgical therapy of osteonecrosis of the jaw: Associated risk factors in aged patients. *Clin. Interv. Aging* **2019**, *14*, 797. [CrossRef] [PubMed]
2. Chen, Z.; Chen, L.; Liu, R.; Lin, Y.; Chen, S.; Lu, S.; Lin, Z.; Chen, Z.; Wu, C.; Xiao, Y. The osteoimmunomodulatory property of a barrier collagen membrane and its manipulation via coating nanometer-sized bioactive glass to improve guided bone regeneration. *Biomater. Sci.* **2018**, *6*, 1007–1019. [CrossRef] [PubMed]
3. Scantlebury, T.V. 1982–1992: A decade of technology development for guided tissue regeneration. *J. Periodontol.* **1993**, *64*, 1129–1137. [CrossRef] [PubMed]
4. Soldatos, N.K.; Stylianou, P.; Koidou, V.P.; Angelov, N.; Yukna, R.; Romanos, G.E. Limitations and options using resorbable versus nonresorbable membranes for successful guided bone regeneration. *Quintessence Int.* **2017**, *48*, 131–147. [CrossRef]
5. Rakhmatia, Y.D.; Ayukawa, Y.; Furuhashi, A.; Koyano, K. Current barrier membranes: Titanium mesh and other membranes for guided bone regeneration in dental applications. *J. Prosthodont. Res.* **2013**, *57*, 3–14. [CrossRef]
6. Dimitriou, R.; Mataliotakis, G.I.; Calori, G.M.; Giannoudis, P.V. The role of barrier membranes for guided bone regeneration and restoration of large bone defects: Current experimental and clinical evidence. *BMC Med.* **2012**, *10*, 81. [CrossRef]
7. Elgali, I.; Omar, O.; Dahlin, C.; Thomsen, P. Guided bone regeneration: Materials and biological mechanisms revisited. *Eur. J. Oral Sci.* **2017**, *125*, 315–337. [CrossRef]
8. Trobos, M.; Juhlin, A.; Shah, F.A.; Hoffman, M.; Sahlin, H.; Dahlin, C. In vitro evaluation of barrier function against oral bacteria of dense and expanded polytetrafluoroethylene (PTFE) membranes for guided bone regeneration. *Clin. Implant. Dent. Relat. Res.* **2018**, *20*, 738–748. [CrossRef]
9. Miron, R.J.; Fujioka-Kobayashi, M.; Buser, D.; Zhang, Y.; Bosshardt, D.D.; Sculean, A. Combination of Collagen Barrier Membrane with Enamel Matrix Derivative-Liquid Improves Osteoblast Adhesion and Differentiation. *Int. J. Oral Maxillofac. Implant.* **2017**, *32*, 196–203. [CrossRef]
10. Li, W.; Ding, Y.; Yu, S.; Yao, Q.; Boccaccini, A.R. Multifunctional Chitosan-45S5 Bioactive Glass-Poly(3-hydroxybutyrate-co-3-hydroxyvalerate) Microsphere Composite Membranes for Guided Tissue/Bone Regeneration. *ACS Appl. Mater. Interfaces* **2015**, *7*, 20845–20854. [CrossRef]
11. Alauddin, M.S.; Abdul Hayei, N.A.; Sabarudin, M.A.; Mat Baharin, N.H. Barrier Membrane in Regenerative Therapy: A Narrative Review. *Membranes* **2022**, *12*, 444. [CrossRef] [PubMed]
12. Chen, X.; Zhu, L.; Liu, H.; Wen, W.; Li, H.; Zhou, C.; Luo, B. Biomineralization guided by polydopamine-modifed poly (L-lactide) fibrous membrane for promoted osteoconductive activity. *Biomed. Mater.* **2019**, *14*, 055005. [CrossRef] [PubMed]
13. Pandey, A.; Yang, T.S.; Yang, T.I.; Belem, W.F.; Teng, N.C.; Chen, I.W.; Huang, C.S.; Kareiva, A.; Yang, J.C. An Insight into Nano Silver Fluoride-Coated Silk Fibroin Bioinspired Membrane Properties for Guided Tissue Regeneration. *Polymers* **2021**, *13*, 2659. [CrossRef] [PubMed]

14. Chu, C.; Deng, J.; Man, Y.; Qu, Y. Evaluation of nanohydroxyapaptite (nano-HA) coated epigallocatechin-3-gallate (EGCG) cross-linked collagen membranes. *Mater. Sci. Eng. C Mater. Biol. Appl.* **2017**, *78*, 258–264. [CrossRef]
15. Dau, M.; Volprich, L.; Grambow, E.; Vollmar, B.; Frerich, B.; Al-Nawas, B.; Kämmerer, P.W. Collagen membranes of dermal and pericardial origin—In vivo evolvement of vascularization over time. *J. Biomed. Mater. Res. Part A* **2020**, *108*, 2368–2378. [CrossRef]
16. Dubus, M.; Rammal, H.; Alem, H.; Bercu, N.B.; Royaud, I.; Quilès, F.; Boulmedais, F.; Gangloff, S.C.; Mauprivez, C.; Kerdjoudj, H. Boosting mesenchymal stem cells regenerative activities on biopolymers-calcium phosphate functionalized collagen membrane. *Colloids Surf. B Biointerfaces* **2019**, *181*, 671–679. [CrossRef]
17. Yang, L.; Zhou, J.; Yu, K.; Yang, S.; Sun, T.; Ji, Y.; Xiong, Z.; Guo, X. Surface modified small intestinal submucosa membrane manipulates sequential immunomodulation coupled with enhanced angio-and osteogenesis towards ameliorative guided bone regeneration. *Mater. Sci. Eng. C* **2021**, *119*, 111641. [CrossRef]
18. Higuchi, J.; Fortunato, G.; Woźniak, B.; Chodara, A.; Domaschke, S.; Męczyńska-Wielgosz, S.; Kruszewski, M.; Dommann, A.; Łojkowski, W. Polymer membranes sonocoated and electrosprayed with nano-hydroxyapatite for periodontal tissues regeneration. *Nanomaterials* **2019**, *9*, 1625. [CrossRef]
19. Van, T.T.T.; Makkar, P.; Farwa, U.; Lee, B.-T. Development of a novel polycaprolactone based composite membrane for periodontal regeneration using spin coating technique. *J. Biomater. Sci. Polym. Ed.* **2022**, *33*, 783–800. [CrossRef]
20. Torres-Lagares, D.; Castellanos-Cosano, L.; Serrera-Figallo, M.Á.; García-García, F.J.; López-Santos, C.; Barranco, A.; Rodriguez-Gonzalez Elipe, A.; Rivera-Jiménez, C.; Gutiérrez-Pérez, J.-L. In vitro and in vivo study of poly (lactic–co–glycolic)(plga) membranes treated with oxygen plasma and coated with nanostructured hydroxyapatite ultrathin films for guided bone regeneration processes. *Polymers* **2017**, *9*, 410. [CrossRef]
21. Torres-Lagares, D.; Castellanos-Cosano, L.; Serrera-Figallo, M.-A.; López-Santos, C.; Barranco, A.; Rodríguez-González-Elipe, A.; Gutierrez-Perez, J.-L. In Vitro Comparative Study of Oxygen Plasma Treated Poly (Lactic–Co–Glycolic)(PLGA) Membranes and Supported Nanostructured Oxides for Guided Bone Regeneration Processes. *Materials* **2018**, *11*, 752. [CrossRef] [PubMed]
22. Byun, S.H.; Lim, H.K.; Kim, S.M.; Lee, S.M.; Kim, H.E.; Lee, J.H. The Bioresorption and Guided Bone Regeneration of Absorbable Hydroxyapatite-Coated Magnesium Mesh. *J. Craniofac. Surg.* **2017**, *28*, 518–523. [CrossRef] [PubMed]
23. Nguyen, T.T.; Jang, Y.S.; Kim, Y.K.; Kim, S.Y.; Lee, M.H.; Bae, T.S. Osteogenesis-Related Gene Expression and Guided Bone Regeneration of a Strontium-Doped Calcium-Phosphate-Coated Titanium Mesh. *ACS Biomater. Sci. Eng.* **2019**, *5*, 6715–6724. [CrossRef] [PubMed]
24. Shi, R.; Ye, J.; Li, W.; Zhang, J.; Li, J.; Wu, C.; Xue, J.; Zhang, L. Infection-responsive electrospun nanofiber mat for antibacterial guided tissue regeneration membrane. *Mater. Sci. Eng. C Mater. Biol. Appl.* **2019**, *100*, 523–534. [CrossRef] [PubMed]
25. Terzopoulou, Z.; Baciu, D.; Gounari, E.; Steriotis, T.; Charalambopoulou, G.; Tzetzis, D.; Bikiaris, D. Composite Membranes of Poly(ε-caprolactone) with Bisphosphonate-Loaded Bioactive Glasses for Potential Bone Tissue Engineering Applications. *Molecules* **2019**, *24*, 3067. [CrossRef]
26. Lian, M.; Sun, B.; Qiao, Z.; Zhao, K.; Zhou, X.; Zhang, Q.; Zou, D.; He, C.; Zhang, X. Bi-layered electrospun nanofibrous membrane with osteogenic and antibacterial properties for guided bone regeneration. *Colloids Surf. B Biointerfaces* **2019**, *176*, 219–229. [CrossRef]
27. Castillo-Dalí, G.; Castillo-Oyagüe, R.; Batista-Cruzado, A.; López-Santos, C.; Rodríguez-González-Elipe, A.; Saffar, J.L.; Lynch, C.D.; Gutiérrez-Pérez, J.L.; Torres-Lagares, D. Reliability of new poly (lactic-co-glycolic acid) membranes treated with oxygen plasma plus silicon dioxide layers for pre-prosthetic guided bone regeneration processes. *Med. Oral. Patol. Oral. Cir. Bucal.* **2017**, *22*, e242–e250. [CrossRef]
28. Lee, J.; Lee, J.; Lee, S.; Ahmad, T.; Madhurakkat Perikamana, S.K.; Kim, E.M.; Lee, S.W.; Shin, H. Bioactive membrane immobilized with lactoferrin for modulation of bone regeneration and inflammation. *Tissue Eng. Part A* **2020**, *26*, 1243–1258. [CrossRef]
29. Hasani-Sadrabadi, M.M.; Sarrion, P.; Nakatsuka, N.; Young, T.D.; Taghdiri, N.; Ansari, S.; Aghaloo, T.; Li, S.; Khademhosseini, A.; Weiss, P.S. Hierarchically patterned polydopamine-containing membranes for periodontal tissue engineering. *ACS Nano* **2019**, *13*, 3830–3838. [CrossRef]
30. Wang, Y.; Zhan, L.; Zhang, X.; Wu, R.; Liao, L.; Wei, J. Silver Nanoparticles Coated Poly(L-Lactide) Electrospun Membrane for Implant Associated Infections Prevention. *Front Pharm.* **2020**, *11*, 431. [CrossRef]
31. Liu, X.; Chen, W.; Shao, B.; Zhang, X.; Wang, Y.; Zhang, S.; Wu, W. Mussel patterned with 4D biodegrading elastomer durably recruits regenerative macrophages to promote regeneration of craniofacial bone. *Biomaterials* **2021**, *276*, 120998. [CrossRef] [PubMed]
32. Xu, Y.; Zhao, S.; Weng, Z.; Zhang, W.; Wan, X.; Cui, T.; Ye, J.; Liao, L.; Wang, X. Jelly-Inspired Injectable Guided Tissue Regeneration Strategy with Shape Auto-Matched and Dual-Light-Defined Antibacterial/Osteogenic Pattern Switch Properties. *ACS Appl. Mater. Interfaces* **2020**, *12*, 54497–54506. [CrossRef] [PubMed]
33. Ejeian, F.; Razmjou, A.; Nasr-Esfahani, M.H.; Mohammad, M.; Karamali, F.; Warkiani, M.E.; Asadnia, M.; Chen, V. ZIF-8 modified polypropylene membrane: A biomimetic cell culture platform with a view to the improvement of guided bone regeneration. *Int. J. Nanomed.* **2020**, *15*, 10029. [CrossRef] [PubMed]
34. van Oirschot, B.A.; Jansen, J.A.; van de Ven, C.J.; Geven, E.J.; Gossen, J.A. Evaluation of collagen membranes coated with testosterone and alendronate to improve guided bone regeneration in mandibular bone defects in minipigs. *J. Oral Maxillofac. Res.* **2020**, *11*, e4. [CrossRef] [PubMed]
35. Van De Ven, C.J.J.M.; Bakker, N.E.C.; Link, D.P.; Geven, E.J.W.; Gossen, J.A. Sustained release of ancillary amounts of testosterone and alendronate from PLGA coated pericard membranes and implants to improve bone healing. *PLoS ONE* **2021**, *16*, e0251864. [CrossRef]

36. Porrelli, D.; Mardirossian, M.; Musciacchio, L.; Pacor, M.; Berton, F.; Crosera, M.; Turco, G. Antibacterial Electrospun Polycaprolactone Membranes Coated with Polysaccharides and Silver Nanoparticles for Guided Bone and Tissue Regeneration. *ACS Appl. Mater. Interfaces* **2021**, *13*, 17255–17267. [CrossRef]
37. Guo, Y.; Yu, Y.; Han, L.; Ma, S.; Zhao, J.; Chen, H.; Yang, Z.; Zhang, F.; Xia, Y.; Zhou, Y. Biocompatibility and osteogenic activity of guided bone regeneration membrane based on chitosan-coated magnesium alloy. *Mater. Sci. Eng. C Mater. Biol. Appl.* **2019**, *100*, 226–235. [CrossRef]
38. Kapa, B.P.; Sowmya, N.K.; Gayathri, G.V.; Mehta, D.S. Coronally advanced flap combined with sticky bone and i-PRF-coated collagen membrane to treat single maxillary gingival recessions: Case series. *Clin. Adv. Periodontics* **2021**. [CrossRef]
39. Ikeda, Y.; Holcroft, J.; Ikeda, E.; Ganss, B. Amelotin Promotes Mineralization and Adhesion in Collagen-Based Systems. *Cell. Mol. Bioeng.* **2022**, *15*, 245–254. [CrossRef]
40. Silva, E.C.; Omonte, S.V.; Martins, A.G.; de Castro, H.H.; Gomes, H.E.; Zenóbio, É.G.; de Oliveira, P.A.; Horta, M.C.; Souza, P.E. Hyaluronic acid on collagen membranes: An experimental study in rats. *Arch. Oral Biol.* **2017**, *73*, 214–222. [CrossRef]
41. Hwang, C.; Park, S.; Kang, I.-G.; Kim, H.-E.; Han, C.-M. Tantalum-coated polylactic acid fibrous membranes for guided bone regeneration. *Mater. Sci. Eng. C* **2020**, *115*, 111112. [CrossRef] [PubMed]
42. Chen, P.; Wu, Z.; Leung, A.; Chen, X.; Landao-Bassonga, E.; Gao, J.; Chen, L.; Zheng, M.; Yao, F.; Yang, H. Fabrication of a silver nanoparticle-coated collagen membrane with anti-bacterial and anti-inflammatory activities for guided bone regeneration. *Biomed. Mater.* **2018**, *13*, 065014. [CrossRef] [PubMed]
43. Zhao, D.; Dong, H.; Niu, Y.; Fan, W.; Jiang, M.; Li, K.; Wei, Q.; Palin, W.M.; Zhang, Z. Electrophoretic deposition of novel semi-permeable coatings on 3D-printed Ti-Nb alloy meshes for guided alveolar bone regeneration. *Dent. Mater.* **2022**, *38*, 431–443. [CrossRef] [PubMed]
44. Boda, S.K.; Fischer, N.G.; Ye, Z.; Aparicio, C. Dual oral tissue adhesive nanofiber membranes for pH-responsive delivery of antimicrobial peptides. *Biomacromolecules* **2020**, *21*, 4945–4961. [CrossRef] [PubMed]
45. Tasiopoulos, C.P.; Petronis, S.; Sahlin, H.; Hedhammar, M. Surface functionalization of PTFE membranes intended for guided bone regeneration using recombinant spider silk. *ACS Appl. Bio Mater.* **2019**, *3*, 577–583. [CrossRef] [PubMed]
46. Choy, S.; Lam, D.V.; Lee, S.M.; Hwang, D.S. Prolonged Biodegradation and Improved Mechanical Stability of Collagen via Vapor-Phase Ti Stitching for Long-Term Tissue Regeneration. *ACS Appl. Mater. Interfaces* **2019**, *11*, 38440–38447. [CrossRef]
47. Zhang, H.Y.; Jiang, H.B.; Kim, J.E.; Zhang, S.; Kim, K.M.; Kwon, J.S. Bioresorbable magnesium-reinforced PLA membrane for guided bone/tissue regeneration. *J. Mech. Behav. Biomed. Mater.* **2020**, *112*, 104061. [CrossRef]
48. De Marco, P.; Zara, S.; De Colli, M.; Radunovic, M.; Lazović, V.; Ettorre, V.; Di Crescenzo, A.; Piattelli, A.; Cataldi, A.; Fontana, A. Graphene oxide improves the biocompatibility of collagen membranes in an in vitro model of human primary gingival fibroblasts. *Biomed. Mater.* **2017**, *12*, 055005. [CrossRef]
49. Fernandes, R.C.; Damasceno, M.I.; Pimentel, G.; Mendonça, J.S.; Gelfuso, M.V.; da Silva Pereira, S.R.L.; Passos, V.F. Development of a membrane for guided tissue regeneration: An in vitro study. *Indian J. Dent. Res.* **2020**, *31*, 763–767. [CrossRef]
50. Steigmann, L.; Jung, O.; Kieferle, W.; Stojanovic, S.; Proehl, A.; Görke, O.; Emmert, S.; Najman, S.; Barbeck, M.; Rothamel, D. Biocompatibility and Immune Response of a Newly Developed Volume-Stable Magnesium-Based Barrier Membrane in Combination with a PVD Coating for Guided Bone Regeneration (GBR). *Biomedicines* **2020**, *8*, 636. [CrossRef]
51. Toyama, N.; Tsuchiya, S.; Kamio, H.; Okabe, K.; Kuroda, K.; Okido, M.; Hibi, H. The effect of macrophages on an atmospheric pressure plasma-treated titanium membrane with bone marrow stem cells in a model of guided bone regeneration. *J. Mater. Sci. Mater. Med.* **2020**, *31*, 1–9. [CrossRef] [PubMed]
52. Zafar, M.S.; Fareed, M.A.; Riaz, S.; Latif, M.; Habib, S.R.; Khurshid, Z. Customized Therapeutic Surface Coatings for Dental Implants. *Coatings* **2020**, *10*, 568. [CrossRef]
53. Jeong, J.; Kim, J.H.; Shim, J.H.; Hwang, N.S.; Heo, C.Y. Bioactive calcium phosphate materials and applications in bone regeneration. *Biomater. Res.* **2019**, *23*, 4. [CrossRef] [PubMed]
54. Riddle, R.C.; Taylor, A.F.; Genetos, D.C.; Donahue, H.J. MAP kinase and calcium signaling mediate fluid flow-induced human mesenchymal stem cell proliferation. *Am. J. Physiol.-Cell Physiol.* **2006**, *290*, C776–C784. [CrossRef]
55. Liu, D.; Genetos, D.C.; Shao, Y.; Geist, D.J.; Li, J.; Ke, H.Z.; Turner, C.H.; Duncan, R.L. Activation of extracellular-signal regulated kinase (ERK1/2) by fluid shear is Ca^{2+}-and ATP-dependent in MC3T3-E1 osteoblasts. *Bone* **2008**, *42*, 644–652. [CrossRef]
56. Danciu, T.E.; Adam, R.M.; Naruse, K.; Freeman, M.R.; Hauschka, P.V. Calcium regulates the PI3K-Akt pathway in stretched osteoblasts. *FEBS Lett.* **2003**, *536*, 193–197. [CrossRef]
57. Julien, M.; Khoshniat, S.; Lacreusette, A.; Gatius, M.; Bozec, A.; Wagner, E.F.; Wittrant, Y.; Masson, M.; Weiss, P.; Beck, L. Phosphate-dependent regulation of MGP in osteoblasts: Role of ERK1/2 and Fra-1. *J. Bone Miner. Res.* **2009**, *24*, 1856–1868. [CrossRef]
58. Tada, H.; Nemoto, E.; Foster, B.L.; Somerman, M.J.; Shimauchi, H. Phosphate increases bone morphogenetic protein-2 expression through cAMP-dependent protein kinase and ERK1/2 pathways in human dental pulp cells. *Bone* **2011**, *48*, 1409–1416. [CrossRef]
59. Hornez, J.C.; Chai, F.; Monchau, F.; Blanchemain, N.; Descamps, M.; Hildebrand, H.F. Biological and physico-chemical assessment of hydroxyapatite (HA) with different porosity. *Biomol. Eng.* **2007**, *24*, 505–509. [CrossRef]
60. Müller, P.; Bulnheim, U.; Diener, A.; Lüthen, F.; Teller, M.; Klinkenberg, E.D.; Neumann, H.G.; Nebe, B.; Liebold, A.; Steinhoff, G. Calcium phosphate surfaces promote osteogenic differentiation of mesenchymal stem cells. *J. Cell. Mol. Med.* **2008**, *12*, 281–291. [CrossRef]
61. Yoshikawa, H.; Myoui, A. Bone tissue engineering with porous hydroxyapatite ceramics. *J. Artif. Organs.* **2005**, *8*, 131–136. [CrossRef] [PubMed]

62. Fernandes, H.R.; Gaddam, A.; Rebelo, A.; Brazete, D.; Stan, G.E.; Ferreira, J.M.F. Bioactive Glasses and Glass-Ceramics for Healthcare Applications in Bone Regeneration and Tissue Engineering. *Materials* **2018**, *11*, 2530. [CrossRef] [PubMed]
63. Hench, L.L.; Polak, J.M. Third-generation biomedical materials. *Science* **2002**, *295*, 1014–1017. [CrossRef] [PubMed]
64. Hench, L.L.; Roki, N.; Fenn, M.B. Bioactive glasses: Importance of structure and properties in bone regeneration. *J. Mol. Struct.* **2014**, *1073*, 24–30. [CrossRef]
65. Day, R.M. Bioactive glass stimulates the secretion of angiogenic growth factors and angiogenesis in vitro. *Tissue Eng.* **2005**, *11*, 768–777. [CrossRef]
66. Monsalve, M.; Ageorges, H.; Lopez, E.; Vargas, F.; Bolivar, F. Bioactivity and mechanical properties of plasma-sprayed coatings of bioglass powders. *Surf. Coat. Technol.* **2013**, *220*, 60–66. [CrossRef]
67. Xue, B.; Guo, L.; Chen, X.; Fan, Y.; Ren, X.; Li, B.; Ling, Y.; Qiang, Y. Electrophoretic deposition and laser cladding of bioglass coating on Ti. *J. Alloys Compd.* **2017**, *710*, 663–669. [CrossRef]
68. Andrée, L.; Barata, D.; Sutthavas, P.; Habibovic, P.; van Rijt, S. Guiding mesenchymal stem cell differentiation using mesoporous silica nanoparticle-based films. *Acta Biomater.* **2019**, *96*, 557–567. [CrossRef]
69. El Yakhlifi, S.; Ball, V. Polydopamine as a stable and functional nanomaterial. *Colloids. Surf. B Biointerfaces* **2020**, *186*, 110719. [CrossRef]
70. Lee, H.; Dellatore, S.M.; Miller, W.M.; Messersmith, P.B. Mussel-inspired surface chemistry for multifunctional coatings. *Science* **2007**, *318*, 426–430. [CrossRef]
71. Ryu, J.; Ku, S.H.; Lee, H.; Park, C.B. Mussel-inspired polydopamine coating as a universal route to hydroxyapatite crystallization. *Adv. Funct. Mater.* **2010**, *20*, 2132–2139. [CrossRef]
72. Batul, R.; Tamanna, T.; Khaliq, A.; Yu, A. Recent progress in the biomedical applications of polydopamine nanostructures. *Biomater. Sci.* **2017**, *5*, 1204–1229. [CrossRef] [PubMed]
73. Ryu, J.H.; Messersmith, P.B.; Lee, H. Polydopamine surface chemistry: A decade of discovery. *ACS Appl. Mater. Interfaces* **2018**, *10*, 7523–7540. [CrossRef] [PubMed]
74. Liu, R.; Guo, Y.; Odusote, G.; Qu, F.; Priestley, R.D. Core–shell Fe_3O_4 polydopamine nanoparticles serve multipurpose as drug carrier, catalyst support and carbon adsorbent. *ACS Appl. Mater. Interfaces* **2013**, *5*, 9167–9171. [CrossRef] [PubMed]
75. Cui, Y.; Yan, Y.; Such, G.K.; Liang, K.; Ochs, C.J.; Postma, A.; Caruso, F. Immobilization and intracellular delivery of an anticancer drug using mussel-inspired polydopamine capsules. *Biomacromolecules* **2012**, *13*, 2225–2228. [CrossRef]
76. Li, Y.; Wang, J.; Ren, F.; Zhang, W.; Zhang, H.; Zhao, L.; Zhang, M.; Cui, W.; Wang, X.; Guo, H. Lactoferrin promotes osteogenesis through TGF-β receptor II binding in osteoblasts and activation of canonical TGF-β signaling in MC3T3-E1 cells and C57BL/6J mice. *J. Nutr.* **2018**, *148*, 1285–1292. [CrossRef]
77. Hering, N.A.; Luettig, J.; Krug, S.M.; Wiegand, S.; Gross, G.; van Tol, E.A.; Schulzke, J.D.; Rosenthal, R. Lactoferrin protects against intestinal inflammation and bacteria-induced barrier dysfunction in vitro. *Ann. N. Y. Acad. Sci.* **2017**, *1405*, 177–188. [CrossRef]
78. Anastasilakis, A.D.; Polyzos, S.A.; Yavropoulou, M.P.; Makras, P. Combination and sequential treatment in women with postmenopausal osteoporosis. *Expert Opin. Pharmacother.* **2020**, *21*, 477–490. [CrossRef]
79. Mohamad, N.-V.; Soelaiman, I.-N.; Chin, K.-Y. A concise review of testosterone and bone health. *Clin. Interv. Aging* **2016**, *11*, 1317–1324. [CrossRef]
80. Suh, S.; Park, M.K. Glucocorticoid-induced diabetes mellitus: An important but overlooked problem. *Endocrinol. Metab.* **2017**, *32*, 180–189. [CrossRef]
81. Riaz Rajoka, M.S.; Mehwish, H.M.; Wu, Y.; Zhao, L.; Arfat, Y.; Majeed, K.; Anwaar, S. Chitin/chitosan derivatives and their interactions with microorganisms: A comprehensive review and future perspectives. *Crit. Rev. Biotechnol.* **2020**, *40*, 365–379. [CrossRef] [PubMed]
82. Blatt, S.; Burkhardt, V.; Kämmerer, P.W.; Pabst, A.M.; Sagheb, K.; Heller, M.; Al-Nawas, B.; Schiegnitz, E. Biofunctionalization of porcine-derived collagen matrices with platelet rich fibrin: Influence on angiogenesis in vitro and in vivo. *Clin. Oral Investig.* **2020**, *24*, 3425–3436. [CrossRef] [PubMed]
83. Venezia, E.; Goldstein, M.; Boyan, B.D.; Schwartz, Z. The use of enamel matrix derivative in the treatment of periodontal defects: A literature review and meta-analysis. *Crit. Rev. Oral Biol. Med. Off. Publ. Am. Assoc. Oral Biol.* **2004**, *15*, 382–402. [CrossRef] [PubMed]
84. Iwasaki, K.; Bajenova, E.; Somogyi-Ganss, E.; Miller, M.; Nguyen, V.; Nourkeyhani, H.; Gao, Y.; Wendel, M.; Ganss, B. Amelotin–a Novel Secreted, Ameloblast-specific Protein. *J. Dent. Res.* **2005**, *84*, 1127–1132. [CrossRef] [PubMed]
85. Nakayama, Y.; Holcroft, J.; Ganss, B. Enamel Hypomineralization and Structural Defects in Amelotin-deficient Mice. *J. Dent. Res.* **2015**, *94*, 697–705. [CrossRef]
86. Abbarin, N.; San Miguel, S.; Holcroft, J.; Iwasaki, K.; Ganss, B. The enamel protein amelotin is a promoter of hydroxyapatite mineralization. *J. Bone Miner. Res.* **2015**, *30*, 775–785. [CrossRef]
87. Price, R.D.; Berry, M.G.; Navsaria, H.A. Hyaluronic acid: The scientific and clinical evidence. *J. Plast. Reconstr. Aesthet. Surg.* **2007**, *60*, 1110–1119. [CrossRef]
88. Fraser, J.R.; Laurent, T.C.; Laurent, U.B. Hyaluronan: Its nature, distribution, functions and turnover. *J. Intern. Med.* **1997**, *242*, 27–33. [CrossRef]
89. Campo, G.M.; Avenoso, A.; D'Ascola, A.; Prestipino, V.; Scuruchi, M.; Nastasi, G.; Calatroni, A.; Campo, S. Hyaluronan differently modulates TLR-4 and the inflammatory response in mouse chondrocytes. *Biofactors* **2012**, *38*, 69–76. [CrossRef]
90. Jiang, D.; Liang, J.; Noble, P.W. Hyaluronan in tissue injury and repair. *Annu. Rev. Cell Dev. Biol.* **2007**, *23*, 435–461. [CrossRef]

91. Park, D.; Kim, Y.; Kim, H.; Kim, K.; Lee, Y.-S.; Choe, J.; Hahn, J.-H.; Lee, H.; Jeon, J.; Choi, C. Hyaluronic acid promotes angiogenesis by inducing RHAMM-TGFβ receptor interaction via CD44-PKCδ. *Mol. Cells* **2012**, *33*, 563–574. [CrossRef] [PubMed]
92. Iturriaga, V.; Bornhardt, T.; Manterola, C.; Brebi, P. Effect of hyaluronic acid on the regulation of inflammatory mediators in osteoarthritis of the temporomandibular joint: A systematic review. *Int. J. Oral Maxillofac. Surg.* **2017**, *46*, 590–595. [CrossRef] [PubMed]
93. Dahiya, P.; Kamal, R. Hyaluronic acid: A boon in periodontal therapy. *N. Am. J. Med. Sci.* **2013**, *5*, 309. [CrossRef] [PubMed]
94. Wang, N.; Li, H.; Wang, J.; Chen, S.; Ma, Y.; Zhang, Z. Study on the anticorrosion, biocompatibility, and osteoinductivity of tantalum decorated with tantalum oxide nanotube array films. *ACS Appl. Mater. Interfaces* **2012**, *4*, 4516–4523. [CrossRef] [PubMed]
95. Wang, Q.; Qiao, Y.; Cheng, M.; Jiang, G.; He, G.; Chen, Y.; Zhang, X.; Liu, X. Tantalum implanted entangled porous titanium promotes surface osseointegration and bone ingrowth. *Sci. Rep.* **2016**, *6*, 26248. [CrossRef]
96. Balla, V.K.; Banerjee, S.; Bose, S.; Bandyopadhyay, A. Direct laser processing of a tantalum coating on titanium for bone replacement structures. *Acta Biomater.* **2010**, *6*, 2329–2334. [CrossRef]
97. Burghardt, I.; Lüthen, F.; Prinz, C.; Kreikemeyer, B.; Zietz, C.; Neumann, H.G.; Rychly, J. A dual function of copper in designing regenerative implants. *Biomaterials* **2015**, *44*, 36–44. [CrossRef]
98. Athinarayanan, J.; Periasamy, V.S.; Krishnamoorthy, R.; Alshatwi, A.A. Evaluation of antibacterial and cytotoxic properties of green synthesized Cu(2)O/Graphene nanosheets. *Mater. Sci. Eng. C Mater. Biol. Appl.* **2018**, *93*, 242–253. [CrossRef]
99. Franci, G.; Falanga, A.; Galdiero, S.; Palomba, L.; Rai, M.; Morelli, G.; Galdiero, M. Silver Nanoparticles as Potential Antibacterial Agents. *Molecules* **2015**, *20*, 8856–8874. [CrossRef]
100. Biel, M.A.; Sievert, C.; Usacheva, M.; Teichert, M.; Balcom, J. *Antimicrobial Photodynamic Therapy Treatment of Chronic Recurrent Sinusitis Biofilms*; Wiley Online Library: New York, NY, USA, 2011; pp. 329–334.
101. Kalishwaralal, K.; BarathManiKanth, S.; Pandian, S.R.K.; Deepak, V.; Gurunathan, S. Silver nanoparticles impede the biofilm formation by Pseudomonas aeruginosa and Staphylococcus epidermidis. *Colloids Surf. B Biointerfaces* **2010**, *79*, 340–344. [CrossRef]
102. Mohanty, S.; Mishra, S.; Jena, P.; Jacob, B.; Sarkar, B.; Sonawane, A. An investigation on the antibacterial, cytotoxic, and antibiofilm efficacy of starch-stabilized silver nanoparticles. *Nanomed. Nanotechnol. Biol. Med.* **2012**, *8*, 916–924. [CrossRef] [PubMed]
103. Habash, M.B.; Park, A.J.; Vis, E.C.; Harris, R.J.; Khursigara, C.M. Synergy of silver nanoparticles and aztreonam against Pseudomonas aeruginosa PAO1 biofilms. *Antimicrob. Agents Chemother.* **2014**, *58*, 5818–5830. [CrossRef] [PubMed]
104. Bryaskova, R.; Pencheva, D.; Nikolov, S.; Kantardjiev, T. Synthesis and comparative study on the antimicrobial activity of hybrid materials based on silver nanoparticles (AgNps) stabilized by polyvinylpyrrolidone (PVP). *J. Chem. Biol.* **2011**, *4*, 185–191. [CrossRef] [PubMed]
105. Zafar, M.S.; Al-Samadani, K.H. Potential use of natural silk for bio-dental applications. *J. Taibah. Univ. Med. Sci.* **2014**, *9*, 171–177. [CrossRef]
106. Chung, H.; Kim, T.Y.; Lee, S.Y. Recent advances in production of recombinant spider silk proteins. *Curr. Opin. Biotechnol.* **2012**, *23*, 957–964. [CrossRef]
107. Wohlrab, S.; Spieß, K.; Scheibel, T. Varying surface hydrophobicities of coatings made of recombinant spider silk proteins. *J. Mater. Chem.* **2012**, *22*, 22050–22054. [CrossRef]
108. Mohnen, D. Pectin structure and biosynthesis. *Curr. Opin. Plant Biol.* **2008**, *11*, 266–277. [CrossRef]
109. Sriamornsak, P. Application of pectin in oral drug delivery. *Expert Opin. Drug Deliv.* **2011**, *8*, 1009–1023. [CrossRef]
110. Geim, A.K.; Novoselov, K.S. The rise of graphene. In *Nanoscience and Technology: A Collection of Reviews from Nature Journals*; World Scientific: Singapore, 2010; pp. 11–19.
111. Zuo, P.-P.; Feng, H.-F.; Xu, Z.-Z.; Zhang, L.-F.; Zhang, Y.-L.; Xia, W.; Zhang, W.-Q. Fabrication of biocompatible and mechanically reinforced graphene oxide-chitosan nanocomposite films. *Chem. Cent. J.* **2013**, *7*, 39. [CrossRef]

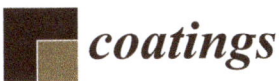

Systematic Review

Titanium Meshes in Guided Bone Regeneration: A Systematic Review

Ricard Aceves-Argemí [1], Elisabet Roca-Millan [1], Beatriz González-Navarro [1,2], Antonio Marí-Roig [2,3], Eugenio Velasco-Ortega [4] and José López-López [2,5,*]

1. Faculty of Medicine and Health Sciences, School of Dentistry, University of Barcelona, 08907 Barcelona, Spain; ricard8aceves@gmail.com (R.A.-A.); erocamil@gmail.com (E.R.-M.); beatrizgonzaleznavarro@gmail.com (B.G.-N.)
2. Oral Health and Masticatory System Group-IDIBELL, Faculty of Medicine and Health Sciences, School of Dentistry, Odontological Hospital University of Barcelona, University of Barcelona, 08907 Barcelona, Spain; amari@bellvitgehospital.cat
3. Department of Maxillofacial Surgery, University Hospital of Bellvitge, 08907 Barcelona, Spain
4. Department of Stomatology, Faculty of Dentistry, University of Seville, 41013 Seville, Spain; evelasco@us.es
5. Department of Odontostomatology, Faculty of Medicine and Health Sciences (Dentistry), Odontological Hospital University of Barcelona, University of Barcelona, 08907 Barcelona, Spain
* Correspondence: jl.lopez@ub.edu

Abstract: The presence of satisfactory bone volume is fundamental for the achievement of osseointegration. This systematic review aims to analyse the use of titanium meshes in guided bone regeneration in terms of bone gain, survival and success rates of implants, and percentages of exposure. An electronic search was conducted Articles were selected from databases in MEDLINE (PubMed), SCOPUS, Scielo, and Cochrane Library databases to identify studies in which bone regeneration was performed through particulate bone and the use of titanium meshes. Twenty-one studies were included in the review. In total, 382 patients, 416 titanium meshes, and 709 implants were evaluated. The average bone gain was 4.3 mm in horizontal width and 4.11 mm in vertical height. The mesh exposure was highly prevalent (28%). The survival rate of 145 simultaneous implants was 99.5%; the survival rate of 507 delayed implants was 99%. The success rate of 105 simultaneous implants was 97%; the success rate of 285 delayed implants was 95.1%. The clinical studies currently available in the literature have shown the predictability of this technique. It has a high risk of soft tissue dehiscence and membrane exposure although the optimal management of membrane exposition permits obtaining a sufficient bone regeneration volume and prevents compromising the final treatment outcome.

Keywords: titanium mesh; bone graft; guided bone regeneration; ridge augmentation

1. Introduction

Satisfactory bone volume is the first condition for obtaining a predictable long-term prognosis in oral implantology. However, some patients may present inadequate bone, which frequently makes difficult the successful outcome of the correct implant placement. Different techniques have been developed to increase bone volume, but at the present time, guided bone regeneration (GBR) represents the gold standard in bone regeneration for implant placement [1,2]. The biological bases of this technique focus on the "PASS" principles: primary closure, angiogenesis, space maintenance, and blood clot stability [3], in other words, this technique focus on the mechanical protection of the blood clot and the isolating of the bone defect, by using a barrier, to facilitate the migration and proliferation of bone-forming cells and to prevent soft tissue colonization inside the bone defect [1,4]. In the last two decades, several membrane designs have been studied. They can be divided into two categories: absorbable and non-resorbable, with different physical and biomaterial properties between them, but all types must have some properties such as

Citation: Aceves-Argemí, R.; Roca-Millan, E.; González-Navarro, B.; Marí-Roig, A.; Velasco-Ortega, E.; López-López, J. Titanium Meshes in Guided Bone Regeneration: A Systematic Review. *Coatings* **2021**, *11*, 316. https://doi.org/10.3390/coatings11030316

Academic Editor: Jun-Beom Park

Received: 21 February 2021
Accepted: 8 March 2021
Published: 10 March 2021

Publisher's Note: MDPI stays neutral with regard to jurisdictional claims in published maps and institutional affiliations.

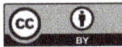

Copyright: © 2021 by the authors. Licensee MDPI, Basel, Switzerland. This article is an open access article distributed under the terms and conditions of the Creative Commons Attribution (CC BY) license (https://creativecommons.org/licenses/by/4.0/).

biocompatibility, tissue integration, space-making, cell selectivity, tissue integration, and clinical manageability [5,6]. The physical and biomaterial properties of the membranes will influence the development of their function, as well as the result of the treatment, therefore, it will be of great importance to know the advantages and disadvantages of each of them [5,6].

The non-resorbable barriers are expanded and dense forms of titanium-reinforced polytetrafluoroethylene membranes (e-PTFE and d-PTFE), the titanium foils, and perforated titanium meshes (preshaped or customized) (Figure 1).

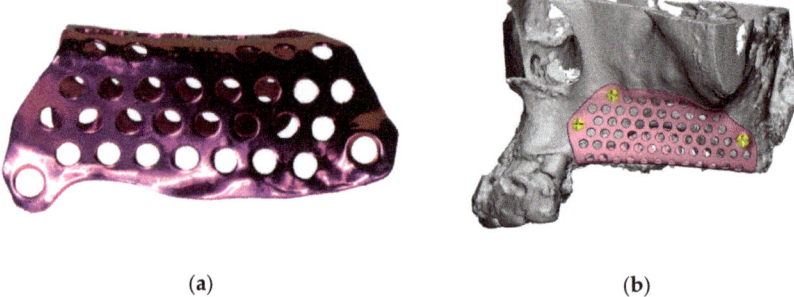

(a)   (b)

Figure 1. (a) Custom-made titanium mesh (AVINENT®® Digital Health); (b) Use of Computer-Aided Design (CAD) and Computer-Aided manufacturing (CAM) to design custom-made devices for guided bone regeneration (GBR).

The biggest disadvantage of these types of membranes is they need to be removed with a second-stage surgical procedure. Despite this, they offer several advantages such as, maintaining the space for a sufficient period of time, providing an effective barrier function in terms of biocompatibility, they are simple to manage and present a reduced risk of long-term complications [7].

In cases where vertical augmentation is desired, or in the presence of severe bone atrophy, the use of more resistant and stable membranes is required. To satisfy these requirements, the e-PTFE membranes were subjected to modifications such as titanium reinforcement that favoured their properties and predictability, or the use of screws in its fixation to improve stability [8]. Thus, the titanium mesh appeared to intend to obtain a balance between the ideal malleability and enough rigidity to accomplish reconstructions of wide bone defects [9].

In the last 8 years, only three reviews about this subject have been conducted [10–12], therefore, the main objective was to assess the use of titanium meshes during guided bone regeneration, the quantity of augmented bone, survival and success rates of implants, complications, and predictability of this surgical technique.

2. Materials and Methods

The systematic review was reported following the Preferred Reporting Items for Systematic Reviews and Meta-Analyses (PRISMA) scale [13]).

2.1. Focused Questions

The following focused questions were formulated:

1. Is the use of titanium mesh in combination with a particulate bone graft (autologous and/or heterologous) a successful technique regarding the quantity of augmented bone?
2. What is the percentage of membrane exposures?
3. What are the implant survival, success, and failure rate when performing this bone regeneration technique in simultaneous or delayed implant placement?

2.2. PICO Question

Bulleted lists look like this:

- P: Patients with partially o total edentulism candidates for GBR.
- I: Bone regeneration through autologous and/or heterologous bone graft and the use of titanium meshes.
- C: Different grafting materials and techniques.
- O: The success rate of this technique regarding the quantity of augmented bone, complications, and predictability of this surgical technique.

2.3. Eligibility Criteria

Inclusion criteria: (i) Studies in which a bone regeneration was performed using particulate bone graft (autologous and/or heterologous) and the use of titanium meshes; (ii) Clinical trials, cohort studies, and case series; (iii) Published in English or Spanish; (iv) Minimum 6 months follow-up period.

Exclusion criteria: (i) Studies performed in vitro or on animals; (ii) Systematic reviews, case reports, and expert opinions; (iii) Studies published before January 2000.

2.4. Information Sources

An electronic search was conducted in MEDLINE (PubMed), SCOPUS, Scielo, and Cochrane Library databases for articles published between 2000 and 2021. References of relevant studies selected were also searched to identify articles with potential inclusion. The last search was performed on 8th January 2021.

2.5. Search Strategy

The following search terms were used:

1. (Titanium mesh [All Fields] AND bone graft [All Fields]).
2. ((Titanium mesh [All Fields] AND (guided bone regeneration [All Fields] OR GBR [All Fields])).
3. (Titanium mesh [All Fields] AND ridge augmentation [All Fields]).

2.6. Study Selection

All articles were reviewed initially by three experts (R.A.-A., E.R.-M., and B.G.-N.). In the event of any discrepancies, these were resolved by J.L.-L.

The first phase of the research consisted of the selection of titles, to eliminate those not concerning our research and eliminate the repeated ones. The second phase consisted of reading the abstract of each article to evaluate some parameters of inclusion. Finally, the full text of all studies selected was obtained.

2.7. Data Collection Process and Items

One reviewer R.A.-A., extracted the data from the selected studies, including characteristics of the study (authors, year of publication, country, and design), sample characteristics (number of patients, mean ages, and number of sites), surgery characteristics (the type of defect, type of surgery performed and materials used) and finally, the post-operatory details and outcomes (follow-up period, percentage of membrane exposures, horizontal/vertical bone regeneration obtained and implant survival, success, and failure rate) which were synthesized in Table 1 and Table 5. A second author (B.G.-N.) verified all the information collected.

The implant success rate was evaluated according to Albrektsson et al. criteria [14]: (i) Absence of subjective complaints such as pain, foreign body sensation, and/or dysesthesia; (ii) Absence of mobility; (iii) Absence of peri-implant radiolucency and infection with pus suppuration; (iv) Marginal bone resorption (MBR) not exceeding 1.5 mm after the first year of loading and up to 0.2 mm yearly thereafter.

2.8. Risk of Bias in Individual Studies

The methodology of the included randomized clinical trials (RCT) was evaluated using the Cochrane Collaboration's risk of bias (RoB 2) tool [15]. The risk of bias for the non-randomized clinical trials (NRCT), was determined using the non-randomized clinical trials of Interventions (ROBINS-I) assessment tool [16]. The risk of bias was classified as "low risk", "unclear risk", and "high risk".

Table 1. Characteristics of the included studies.

Author/Country	Type of Study	"N" M	"N" F	Mean Ages (y)	Number of Sites Mx	Number of Sites Md	Type of Defects	Graft Materials	Second-Stage Surgery (m)	Mesh Exposure (%)	Bone Augmentation (mm) MHA	Bone Augmentation (mm) MVA
Miyamoto et al., 2001/Japan [17]	Case series	16	25	46	29	21	C, V, S	Autologous	6	36	4	8,9
Degidi et al., 2003/Italy [18]	Case series	4	14	47.5	-	-	-	Autologous	4Md 6Mx	0	-	-
Proussaefs et al., 2006/USA [19]	Case series	10	7	50.6	17		C	Autologous + ABB 50:50	8.47	35.3	3.75	2.56
Pinho et al., 2006/Brazil [20]	RCT	10		46.3	10 10	-	V, H	Test: Autologous Control: None	6	50	8.4[1] 8.8[1]	1.4[1] 1.4[1]
Corinaldesi et al., 2007/Italy [21]	NRCT	3 4	3 2	49.3 57.7	3 3	3 3	C	Test: Autologous + BPBM 70:30 Control: Autologous	8–9	-	- -	4 4.16
Pieri et al., 2008/Italy [22]	Prospective study	7	9	49.6	9	10	C	Autologous + ABB 70:30	8–9	5.3	4.16	3.71
Corinaldesi et al., 2009/Italy [23]	Case series	9	15	48.4	27		C	Autologous	8–9	14.8	-	4.9
Torres et al., 2010/Spain [24]	RCT	7 6	9 8	-	27	16	V, H, C	Test: ABB + PRP Control: ABB	6	0 28.5	3.4 3.1	4.1 3.7
Her et al., 2012/South Korea [25]	Case series	11	15	51	9	18	C, H	Autologous + ABB Alloplastic Autologous+Alloplastic	5.7	26	-	-
Lizio et al., 2014/Italy [26]	Case series	2	10	49.1	11	4	C, V	Autologous + ABB 70:30	8–9	80	-	-
Poli et al., 2014/Italy [27]	Case series	8	5	-	11	2	C	Autologous + DBBM 50:50	6	7.68	-	-
Sumida et al., 2014/Japan [28]	NRCT	3 4	10 9	47 48	-	-	-	Autologous + CD Autologous + CMD	6	23.1 7.7	- -	- -
Uehara et al., 2015/Germany [29]	Case series	7	14	47.5	11	12	C, V, S	Autologous + Hydroxyapatite 50:50	3–7	70	-	-
Zita et al., 2016/Portugal [30]	Case series	15	10	54.3	-	-	H	ABB	3–4	24	3.67	-
Bassi et al., 2016/Italy [31]	Case series	1	9	58	0	10	C, H, V	TMAP	6.7	30	8.6	6.1
Ciocca et al., 2018/Italy [32]	Prospective study	3	6	50.2	6	5	V	Autologous + ABB 50:50	6–8	66.6	-	3.8 Md 3.9 Mx
Cucchi et al., 2019/Italy [33]	RCT	20		52	-	-	V	Autologous + Allograft 50:50	9	21.1	-	4.1
Zhang et al., 2019/China [34]	Case series	12		-	16	0	C	ABB	4–8	6.25	3.1	3.61
Atef et al., 2020/Egypt [35]	RCT	10		-	-	-	H	Autologous + ABB 50:50	6	40	3.7	-

Table 1. Cont.

Author/Country	Type of Study	"N" M	"N" F	Mean Ages (y)	Number of Sites Mx	Number of Sites Md	Type of Defects	Graft Materials	Second-Stage Surgery (m)	Mesh Exposure (%)	Bone Augmentation (mm) MHA	Bone Augmentation (mm) MVA
Malik et al., 2020/India [36]	Case series	12	8	48.7	0	20	V	TMAP	6	20	-	4.82
Cucchi et al., 2020/Italy [37]	Case series	5	5	52	5	5	V	Autologous + ABB 50:50	6–9	10	-	4.5

Mx: Maxilla; Md: Mandible; MHA: Mean horizontal augmentation; MVA: Mean vertical augmentation C: Combined; H: Horizontal; V: Vertical; S: Socket; DBBM: Demineralized bovine bone mineral; ABB: Inorganic bovine bone; BPBM: Bovine porous bone protein; TMAP: Thermoplastic mouldable allograft paste. RCT: Randomized clinical trial; NRCT: Non-randomized clinical trial.[1]: Referred to vertical and horizontal bone fill of sockets after tooth extraction; CD: Conventional device; CMD: Custom made device.

3. Results

3.1. Study Selection

A total of 572 articles were identified in the first phase of the research. During the second phase, 94 articles were considered, and after full-text evaluation 16 studies were included in the review. Finally, five articles of interest were obtained through manual research obtaining a total of 21 articles were included in this review [17–37] (Figure 2).

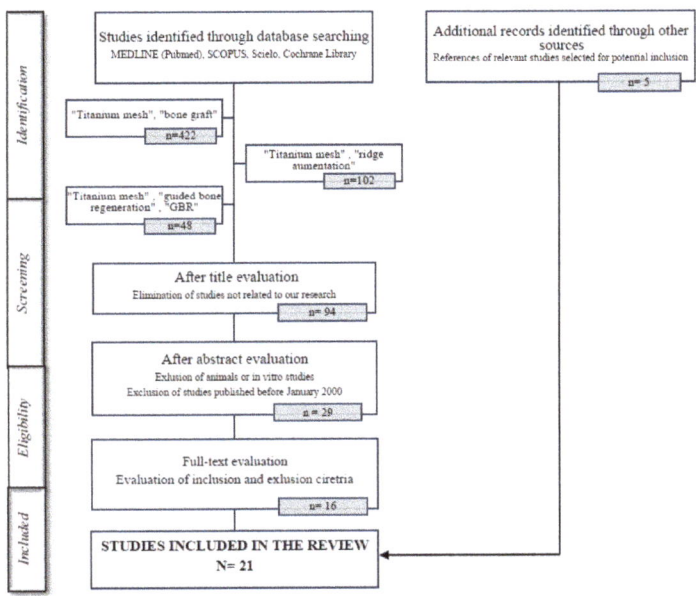

Figure 2. Flow diagram of study inclusion.

3.2. Study Methods and Characteristics

Four studies were RCT [20,24,33,35], 2 were NRCT [21,28], 2 were prospective studies [22,32] and 13 were case series [17–19,23,25–27,29–31,34,36,37] and all of them were published between 2001 and 2021 (Table 1).

The studies were conducted in nine different countries, the total number of patients included was 382 (137 males, 193 females, and 52 non-specified) and a total of 416 titanium meshes.

There were four articles in which the gender was not specified [20,33–35]. The study with a higher number of patients was Miyamoto et al. (N = 41) [17] while the one with fewer patients was Ciocca et al. [29] with a total of nine patients. The mean age was 53.4 and four articles did not specify the mean age [24,27,34,35].

Regarding the characteristics of the surgeries performed, it was quantified the number of sites, and whether if it was in mandible or maxilla. In five studies, the number of sites was not specified [18,28,30,34,35], of which 164 sites belong to the maxilla and 129 to the mandible.

In 16 studies the graft material used was autologous bone; in six of them it was the only material used [17,18,20,21,23,28] (N = 120), and in the other 10 articles, autologous bone was associated with other graft materials such as inorganic bovine bone (ABB) [19,22,25,26,32,35,37] (N = 91), thermoplastic mouldable allograft paste (TMAP) [33] (N = 28), bovine porous bone protein (BPBM) [21] (N = 3), demineralized bovine bone mineral (DBBM) [27] (N = 13) or Hydroxyapatite [29] (N = 21). There were five studies in which autologous bone was not used and the regeneration was performed only with the use of ABB [24,30,34] (N = 67) or TMAP (36,31) (N = 39).

The removal of the mesh and the quantification of bone gains was performed during the second-stage surgery or also called in most studies as healing period, which was performed on average at 6.5 months.

3.3. Quality Assessment and Risk of Bias within Studies

The risk of bias of the RCT is presented in Table 2. Three RTCs were considered as having a low risk of bias even though there were some concerns about the blinding of participants and researchers [24,33,35] and Atef et al. did not report the blinding of outcome assessment and selective outcome reporting, potentially introducing selection bias [35]. One study was considered as having a high risk of bias since there were some concerns about the random sequence generation, the allocation concealment, and the blinding of participants and researchers [20].

Table 2. Risk of Bias of included randomized clinical trials.

Author	Random Sequence Generation	Allocation Concealment	Blinding of Participants and Researchers	Blinding of Outcome Assessment	Incomplete Outcome Data	Selective Outcome Reporting	Other Sources of Bias
Pinho et al., 2006 [20]	?	?	?	L	L	?	L
Torres et al., 2010 [21–24]	L	L	?	L	L	L	L
Cucchi et al., 2019 [33]	L	L	?	L	L	L	L
Atef et al., 2020 [35]	L	L	?	?	L	?	L

L: Low; (?): Unclear; H: High.

Two non-randomized clinical trials were included, and the risk of bias is represented in Table 3. These two articles were considered as having a low risk of bias but there were some concerns about potential bias in the classification of interventions [21,28] and also due to deviations from intended interventions [21].

Table 3. Risk of Bias of included non-randomized clinical trials.

Author	Bias Due to Confounding	Bias in Selection of Participants into the Study	Bias in Classification of Interventions	Bias due to Deviations from Intended Interventions	Bias due to Missing data	Bias in Measurement of Outcomes	Overall Bias
Corinaldesi et al., 2007 [21]	L	L	?	?	L	L	L
Sumida et al., 2015 [28]	L	L	?	L	L	L	L

L: Low; (?): Unclear; H: High.

(The systematic review was reported following the Preferred Reporting Items for Systematic Reviews and Meta-Analyses (PRISMA) scale [13]) with 21 items.

3.4. Characteristics of the Mesh

Different types of meshes were used in the studies, all of them are summarized in Table 4.

Table 4. Characteristics of the meshes used.

Authors	Characteristics of the Mesh Used	Thickness
Miyamoto et al., 2001 [17]	Preshaped titanium mesh (M-TAM, Stryker Leinger GmbH & Co., KG, Freiburg ASTM F-67 Jeil Medical Corp., Seoul, Korea)	0.1 and 0.2 mm thick
Degidi et al., 2003 [18]	Preshaped micromesh (Cortical Mesh, Micronova, Bologna, Italy)	NE
Proussaefs et al., 2006 [19]	Preshaped titanium mesh (Osteo-Tram; OsteoMed)	0.2 mm thick
Pinho et al., 2006 [20]	Preshaped titanium mesh (Frios Boneshield; DENTSPLY Friadent)	NE
Corinaldesi et al., 2007 [21]	Preshaped and trimmed titanium micromesh (ACE surgical supply, Straumann)	0.2 mm thick
Pieri et al., 2008 [22]	Preshaped titanium mesh (Modus 1.5 Mesh, Straumann, Waldenburg, Switzerland)	NE
Corinaldesi et al., 2009 [23]	Preshaped and trimmed titanium mesh (ACE Titanium Micro Mesh, ACE Surgical Supply Company; Modus 0.9 Mesh, Medartis)	0.2 mm thick
Torres et al., 2010 [24]	Preshaped and trimmed titanium mesh	NE
Her et al., 2012 [25]	Preshaped and trimmed titanium mesh (Jeil Medical, Seoul, South Korea)	0.1 mm thick
Lizio et al., 2014 [26]	Titanium mesh (ridge-form; OsteoMed)	0.2 mm thick
Poli et al., 2014 [27]	Preshaped and trimmed titanium mesh (ridge-form; (KLS Martin, Tuttlingen, Germany)	0.2 mm thick
Sumida et al., 2014 [28]	Custom-made titanium mesh (Ace Surgical SupplyCo., Inc. Brockton, MA, USA)	0.5 mm thick
Uehara et al., 2015 [29]	Preshaped and trimmed microtitanium mesh (Striker-Leibinger, Freiburg, Germany)	0.1 mm thick
Zita et al., 2016 [30]	Titanium mesh (i–Gen, MegaGen, Gyeongbuk, Republic of Korea)	NE
Bassi et al., 2016 [31]	Titanium foil (grade 4)	0.2 mm thick
Ciocca et al., 2018 [32]	Custom-made titanium mesh (Electro Optical Systems, Munich, Germany)	0.1 mm
Cucchi et al., 2019 [33]	Preshaped titaium mesh (Trinon Titanium; Karlsruhe, Germany)	NE
Zhang et al., 2019 [34]	L-Shaped titanium mesh; Preshaped and trimmed	0.2 mm thick
Atef et al., 2020 [35]	Preshaped titanium mesh (Bioinnovation, Brazil)	NE
Malik et al., 2020 [36]	Preshaped and trimmed titanium mesh	NE
Cucchi et al., 2020 [37]	Custom-made titanium mesh (3D-Mesh®®, Biotec Srl, Dueville, Vicenza, Italy)	>0.5 mm thick

NE: Not evaluated.

3.5. Bone Gain

The bone gains were quantified using cone-beam computed tomography (CBCT) images. In two studies, width bone gain was quantified [30,35], five studies quantified height bone gain [21,23,33,36,37], six studied both width and height bone gains [17,22,24,29,31,34] and finally 5 works did not quantify any bone gains after the surgery [18,22,26,27,29]. The average bone gains were 4.3 mm in horizontal width (range 3.1 mm performed with ABB to 8.6 mm performed with TMAP) and 4.11 mm in vertical height (range 2.56 mm performed with autologous and ABB 50:50 to 8.9 mm performed only with autologous).

One study performed GBR after tooth removal, to evaluate the prevention of alveolar collapse after tooth extraction, using titanium membrane [20].

Four studies evaluated the histologic and histomorphometric outcomes of GBR from biopsies of the newly regenerated bone [19,21,31,33]. According to Bassi et al. [31], the histological and histomorphometric analysis of the samples demonstrates the effectiveness of GBR employing titanium mesh, as a barrier membrane. Cucchi et al. [33] concluded that the regenerated bone differed from the native bone in terms of trabecular organization, as well as newly formed bone remained immature and very different from the native bone. Proussaefs et al. [19] demonstrated 36.47% of bone formation when the titanium mesh was used in combination with autogenous bone and ABB. Corinaldesi et al. [21] concluded that BPBM (30%) in combination with the autologous bone (70%) yielded similar bone formation patterns as autologous bone alone.

3.6. Mesh Exposure

Except for Corinaldesi et al. [21] all the included studies evaluated the mesh exposure (N = 404), and it proved to be a highly prevalent complication, appearing in 115 cases out of 404 meshes (28%) (range 0% to 80%). Of these 115 exposed meshes, 25 were removed due to more severe complications, and 75 were stabilized and controlled through local hygiene measures.

According to the studies in which the implant was placed simultaneously [18,23,30,33,34] the mesh exposure rate was 14% (13 out of 87). In contrast, in the cases of guide bone regeneration (GBR) and delayed implant placement [17,19,21–25,27,29,31,32,37] the mean mesh exposure rate was 30% (58 out of 187).

3.7. Implant Placement

Apart from performing the alveolar ridge augmentation, there were 16 studies in which dental implants were placed [18,19,21–25,27,29–34,37] (Table 4). The other five studies focused on the bone regeneration process without involving implant placement. The outcomes were studied and summarized in Table 5.

In total, 709 implants were placed and the total prevalence of implant failure in this review was 0.5% (4 implants were lost). The follow-up time after the implant placement was on average of 32 months (range 6 to 96).

In five studies, bone augmentation was performed simultaneously with implant placement (N = 145) [18,23,30,33,34], in the other studies, the implant placement was delayed after 7,1 months on average (N = 564) (range 3 to 10 months) [17,19,21–25,27,29,31,32,37].

The implant success rate was assessed considering at least 6 months from the prosthetic load. The survival rate of 145 simultaneous implants was 99.5%; the survival rate of 507 delayed implants was 99%. The success rate of 105 simultaneous implants was 97%; the success rate of 285 delayed implants was 95.1%. Proussaefs et al. [19] did not specify the survival and success rates and Corinaldesi et al. [21], Torres et al. [24], Zita et al. [30], and Ciocca et al. [32] did not specify the success rate.

The marginal bone resorption (MBR) was evaluated in 6 studies and it was on average of 0.75 mm [19,22–24,30,31,37] (N = 234). There were no statistically significant differences between de MBR observed in the simultaneous implants and delayed implants.

Table 5. Evaluation of characteristics of implant placement.

Author/Country	Implant Placement	Implants Mx	Implants Md	Implant Lost	Bone Loss (mm)	Success Rate (%)	Survival Rate (%)	Follow-up (m)
Miyamoto et al., 2001/Japan [17]	After 6 months	89		1	-	94	92.8	47.5
Degidi et al., 2003/Italy [18]	Simultaneously	50		0	-	100	100	84
Proussaefs et al., 2006/USA [19]	After 9–10 months	36	5	-	0 MBR	-	-	6
Corinaldesi et al., 2007/Italy [21]	After 8–9 months	20	15	0	-	-	100	12
Pieri et al., 2008/Italy [22]	After 8–9 months	21	23	0	1.36 MBR	93.2	100	12
Corinaldesi et al., 2009/Italy [23]	Simultaneously After 8–9 months	20 36		0 0	1.22 MBR 1.26 MBR	96.4	100	36–96
Torres et al., 2010/Spain [24]	After 6 months	97		3	-	-	98.6	24
Her et al., 2012/South Korea [25]	After 5–7 months	27	41	0	-	100	100	6–24
Poli et al., 2014/Italy [27]	After 6 months	16	4	0	1.74 M, 1.91 D	100	100	88
Uehara et al., 2015/Germany [29]	After 6 months	64		1	-	-	98.4	40
Zita et al., 2016/Portugal [30]	Simultaneously	32	8	1	0.43 MBR	-	97.5	12
Bassi et al., 2016/Italy [31]	After 6–7 months	0	18	0	1.17 MBR	88.2	100	12
Ciocca et al., 2018/Italy [32]	After 6–8 months	14	12	0	-	-	100	24
Cucchi et al., 2019/Italy [33]	Simultaneously	0	19	0	0 MBR	100	100	12
Zhang et al., 2019/China [34]	Simultaneously	16	0	0	0.81 V 0.13 H	93.75	100	24
Cucchi et al., 2020/Italy [37]	After 6–9 months	14	12	0	0 MBR	100	100	12

M: Mesial; D: Distal; MBR: Marginal bone resorption; V: Vertical; H: Horizontal.

4. Discussion

From the analysis of the recent published articles, few studies concerning GBR using titanium mesh were published. The present systematic review aimed to evaluate the results reported in the literature evaluating the following aspects: (a) the success rate of this technique regarding the quantity of augmented bone; (b) the complications rate by means of exposure; (c) the implants survival and success rate. The topic was focused on the presence of the titanium meshes used as a physical barrier for ridge reconstruction in partial or total edentulism, preventing soft tissue colonization and allowing osteoprogenitor cells to reach the site and form new bone.

4.1. Bone Gain

The use of non-resorbable titanium meshes allows maintaining the shape between the barrier and the bone defect. Furthermore, the pores allow to maintain vascularization both to the soft tissue and to the bone during the regeneration process and facilitates tissue nutrition [12,38]. Generally, the literature showed that the use of non-resorbable titanium meshes in GBR represent a safe and predictable technique to gain vertical and/or horizontal bone augmentation, in the treatment of small and medium-sized defects around dental implants and prevention of alveolar ridge after tooth extraction [9,20,30,35]. The analysis of the studies included in the present systematic review corroborates this statement, although only six included studies quantified both width and height bone gains [17,19,22,24,31,34]. The histological and histomorphometric analysis also demonstrates the effectiveness of GBR using the titanium mesh, and good capacity of the method to increase bone volume in the distal mandibular atrophies [19,21,31,33]. On the other hand, other authors like Uehara et al. [29] appear more doubtful about the success of this technique. According to their success criteria, only 13 sites were judged as successful with a success rate of 56.6%, emphasizing that, the greatest success rate was obtained at the sites with a shorter span of augmentation.

When comparing the success of this technique with other GBR techniques such as the use of PTFE membranes, results of bone gain did not differ much. Cucchi et al. [39] found that the height bone gain was 4.2 (range 2.7 to 5.8) mm when using PTFE and 4.1 (range 2.6 to 6.3) mm when using a titanium mesh. Sagheb et al. [40], found a height bone gain higher (4.16 and 5.5 mm).

Table 6. Incidence of membrane/barrier exposure in different techniques.

Author	Type of Barrier/Membrane	Exposure Rate (%)
Rasia dal Polo et al. [10]	Titanium mesh	16
Ricci et al. [11]	Titanium mesh	22
Briguglio et al. [12]	Titanium mesh	52
Wessing et al. [41]	Collagen membrane	20
Wessing et al. [41]	Cross-linked membrane	28
Ricci et al. [11]	d-PTFE	17
Roca-Millan et al. [42]	Titanium foils	23

4.2. Mesh Exposure

From the analysis of the complications, the investigation was focused on mesh exposures which was the most usual complication when performing this technique. To prevent premature exposure of the augmented area, all the analysed studies highlighted the necessity to mobilize the flaps to obtain a primary wound closure without tensions. According to the results of this review, the mean rate of mesh exposure was 28%. Other reviews about membrane/mesh exposure were found in the literature (Table 6).

The prevalence of mesh exposure in the cases of GBR and delayed implant placement was higher than when simultaneous implant placement. The reason for this higher incidence might be correlated with "free-end" edentulism and severe vertical ridge resorption, as well as a low number of included cases in the simultaneous placement group.

Some authors propose that to reduce the rate of mesh exposure, consensus protocols are needed, but also more precise customized meshes. Also, the use of resorbable membranes and PRP to prevent the risk of early dehiscence [18,43,44].

Even though the most frequent complication associated with this device is its exposure, according to the results of this review, it is worth noting that this event does not necessarily compromise the final treatment outcome and further complications were avoided using topical application of chlorhexidine gel [19,25].

Comparing to other types of techniques, Garcia et al. [45] found that when GBR is associated with collagen membranes or e-PTFE, the exposure of the membrane may influence bone gain. The sites without exposure achieved 74% more horizontal bone gain than sites with membrane exposure. In all types of GBR, meticulous soft-tissue handling is mandatory to obtain flaps without tension over the membranes, in order that the regenerative tissue can be kept entirely covered. When a titanium mesh is exposed and the grafted bone had been sufficiently stabilized by newly formed bone, the integrity of the hole new bone regeneration can be mostly ensured and avoid superinfection. This is possible due to its pores since they play a crucial role in vascularization of the graft and allows its hygiene [19,23,25].

4.3. Characteristics of the Mesh

Regarding the thickness of the mesh most currently used is 0.2 mm (range 0.1–0.5 mm), since it provides sufficient rigidity to maintain space and protect the graft [34,37]. According to other authors, a titanium mesh should be sufficiently stiff to be able to resist the muscular tensions and the pressure of the surgical flap, but at the same quite manageable to be adapted to the bone defect [10–12,30,34,37].

The external form should be as round as possible to avoid damaging he flap and the surface as smooth as possible to avoid bacterial colonization or infection [10,12,37]. In most of the articles, the authors specify the devices were polished and rounded before placed, to avoid dehiscence and soft tissue ruptures.

4.4. Implant Success and Survival Rates

It has been reported that the survival rates of implants placed in regenerated bone were similar to those described for implants placed into native bone [44,45]. The implant survival rate of the included articles of this review was 99.25% and the implant success rate was 93.35%, similar to other works available in the literature [46,47].

4.5. Limitations

It must be taken into account the heterogeneity in design, data collection methods, and analyses performed across the included studies. Moreover, the lack of RTCs with a large sample is observed. Most of the included articles were case series, and some of them did not report the bone gain obtained.

Despite the differences regarding the surgical protocols (collagen membrane association, different timing of mesh removal, different graft materials) results were similar. Therefore, it was not easy to identify the most successful surgical technique when a titanium mesh is used.

Only four studies performed controlled randomization [20,24,33,35], and in one of them, the implant timing, the follow-up, and survival/success implant rates were not specified [20].

5. Conclusions

Based on the literature presented, it is possible to assess that the use of a titanium mesh in combination with autologous and/or heterologous particulate grafts represent a safe and predictable technique to increase vertical and/or horizontal bone volume in cases of defects in partially edentulous patients, in the treatment of small and medium-sized defects around dental implants and alveolar ridge preservation after tooth extraction.

However, the use of titanium meshes presented disadvantages related to the necessity of the second-stage surgical procedure, with increased patient morbidity and rehabilitation time. Furthermore, it has a high risk of soft tissue dehiscence and membrane exposure.

The membrane exposure rate of this technique reaches 28% of the cases. The optimal management of membrane exposition permits obtaining a sufficient bone regeneration volume and prevents compromising the final treatment outcome.

The implant survival and implant success values are similar to those described for implants placed into the native bone and when performing other GBR techniques. No significant differences were observed between the implant survival and implant success rates between simultaneous and delayed implant placement.

Author Contributions: Conceptualization, R.A.-A. and B.G.-N.; methodology, R.A.-A. and B.G.-N.; validation, R.A.-A., B.G.-N. and J.L.-L.; formal analysis, R.A.-A.; investigation, R.A.-A. and E.R.-M.; resources, J.L.-L.; data curation, R.A.-A., E.R.-M. and J.L.-L.; writing—original draft preparation, R.A.-A. and E.R.-M.; writing—review and editing, R.A.-A.; visualization, B.G.-N. and J.L.-L.; project administration, A.M.-R., E.V.-O. and J.L.-L.; All authors have read and agreed to the published version of the manuscript.

Funding: This research received no external funding.

Institutional Review Board Statement: Not applicable.

Informed Consent Statement: Not applicable.

Data Availability Statement: Data is contained within the article.

Conflicts of Interest: The authors declare no conflict of interest.

References

1. Elgali, I.; Omar, O.; Dahlin, C.; Thomsen, P. Guided bone regeneration: Materials and biological mechanisms revisited. *Eur. J. Oral Sci.* **2017**, *125*, 315–337. [CrossRef]
2. Chiapasco, M.; Casentini, P.; Zaniboni, M. Bone augmentation procedures in implant dentistry. *Int. J. Oral Maxillofac. Implant.* **2009**, *24*, 237–259.
3. Wang, H.L.; Boyapati, L. "PASS" principles for predictable bone regeneration. *Implant. Dent.* **2006**, *15*, 8–17. [CrossRef]
4. Dahlin, C.; Linde, A.; Gottlow, J.; Nyman, S. Healing of bone defects by guided tissue regeneration. *Plast. Reconstr. Surg.* **1988**, *81*, 672–676. [CrossRef] [PubMed]
5. Hämmerle, C.H.; Jung, R.E.; Feloutzis, A. A systematic review of the survival of implants in bone sites augmented with barrier membranes (guided bone regeneration) in partially edentulous patients. *J. Clin. Periodontol.* **2002**, *29*, 226–231. [CrossRef] [PubMed]
6. Scantlebury, T.V. 1982–1992: A decade of technology development for guided tissue regeneration. *J. Periodontol.* **1993**, 1129–1137. [CrossRef]
7. Zhang, J.; Xu, Q.; Huang, C.; Mo, A.; Li, J.; Zuo, Y. Biological properties of an anti-bacterial membrane for guided bone regeneration: An experimental study in rats. *Clin. Oral Implant. Res.* **2010**, *21*, 321–327. [CrossRef] [PubMed]
8. Hämmerle, C.H.; Jung, R.E. Bone augmentation by means of barrier membranes. *Periodontology 2000* **2003**, *33*, 36–53. [CrossRef]
9. Rakhmatia, Y.D.; Ayukawa, Y.; Furuhashi, A.; Koyano, K. Current barrier membranes: Titanium mesh and other membranes for guided bone regeneration in dental applications. *J. Prosthodont. Res.* **2013**, *57*, 3–14. [CrossRef]
10. Ricci, L.; Perrotti, V.; Ravera, L.; Scarano, A.; Piattelli, A.; Iezzi, G. Rehabilitation of deficient alveolar ridges using titanium grids before and simultaneously with implant placement: A systematic review. *J. Periodontol.* **2013**, *84*, 1234–1242. [CrossRef]
11. Rasia-dal Polo, M.; Poli, P.P.; Rancitelli, D.; Beretta, M.; Maiorana, C. Alveolar ridge reconstruction with titanium meshes: A systematic review of the literature. *Med. Oral Patol. Oral Cir. Buccal* **2014**, *19*, e639–e646. [CrossRef] [PubMed]
12. Briguglio, F.; Falcomatà, D.; Marconcini, S.; Fiorillo, L.; Briguglio, R.; Farronato, D. The Use of Titanium Mesh in Guided Bone Regeneration: A Systematic Review. *Int. J. Dent.* **2019**, *2019*, 9065423. [CrossRef] [PubMed]
13. Moher, D.; Liberati, A.; Tetzlaff, J.; Altman, D.G. PRISMA Group. Preferred reporting items for systematic reviews and meta-analyses: The PRISMA statement. *PLoS Med.* **2009**, *6*, e1000097. [CrossRef]
14. Albrektsson, T.; Zarb, G.; Worthington, P.; Eriksson, A.-R. The long-term efficacy of currently used dental implants: A review and proposed criteria of success. *Int. J. Oral Maxillofac. Implant.* **1986**, *1*, 11–25.
15. Sterne, J.A.C.; Savović, J.; Page, M.J.; Elbers, R.G.; Blencowe, N.S.; Boutron, I. RoB 2: A revised tool for assessing risk of bias in randomised trials. *BMJ* **2019**, *366*, l4898. [CrossRef] [PubMed]
16. Sterne, J.A.; Hernán, M.A.; Reeves, B.C.; Savović, J.; Berkman, N.D.; Viswanathan, M. ROBINS-1: A tool for assessing risk of bias in non-randomised studies of interventions. *BMJ* **2016**, *355*, i4919. [CrossRef]
17. Miyamoto, I.; Funaki, K.; Yamauchi, K.; Kodama, T.; Takahashi, T. Alveolar ridge reconstruction with titanium mesh and autogenous particulate bone graft: Computed tomography-based evaluations of augmented bone quality and quantity. *Clin. Implant Dent. Relat. Res.* **2012**, *14*, 304–311. [CrossRef]
18. Degidi, M.; Scarano, A.; Piattelli, A. Regeneration of the alveolar crest using titanium micromesh with autologous bone and a resorbable membrane. *J. Oral Implantol.* **2003**, *29*, 86–90. [CrossRef]
19. Proussaefs, P.; Lozada, J. Use of titanium mesh for staged localized alveolar ridge augmentation: Clinical and histologic-histomorphometric evaluation. *J. Oral Implantol.* **2006**, *32*, 237–247. [CrossRef]
20. Pinho, M.N.; Roriz, V.L.; Novaes, A.B.; Taba, M.; Grisi, M.F.; de Souza, S.L.; Palioto, D.B. Titanium membranes in prevention of alveolar collapse after tooth extraction. *Implant. Dent.* **2006**, *15*, 53–61. [CrossRef]
21. Corinaldesi, G.; Pieri, F.; Marchetti, C.; Fini, M.; Aldini, N.N.; Giardino, R. Histologic and histomorphometric evaluation of alveolar ridge augmentation using bone grafts and titanium micromesh in humans. *J. Periodontol.* **2007**, *78*, 1477–1484. [CrossRef] [PubMed]
22. Pieri, F.; Corinaldesi, G.; Fini, M.; Aldini, N.N.; Giardino, R.; Marchetti, C. Alveolar ridge augmentation with titanium mesh and a combination of autogenous bone and anorganic bovine bone: A 2-year prospective study. *J. Periodontol.* **2008**, *79*, 2093–2103. [CrossRef] [PubMed]
23. Corinaldesi, G.; Pieri, F.; Sapigni, L.; Marchetti, C. Evaluation of survival and success rates of dental implants placed at the time of or after alveolar ridge augmentation with an autogenous mandibular bone graft and titanium mesh: A 3- to 8-year retrospective study. *Int. J. Oral Maxillofac. Implant.* **2009**, *24*, 1119–1128.
24. Torres, J.; Tamimi, F.; Alkhraisat, M.H.; Manchón, A.; Linares, R.; Prados-Frutos, J.C.; Hernández, G.; López Cabarcos, E. Platelet-rich plasma may prevent titanium-mesh exposure in alveolar ridge augmentation with anorganic bovine bone. *J. Clin. Periodontol.* **2010**, *37*, 943–951. [CrossRef] [PubMed]
25. Her, S.; Kang, T.; Fien, M.J. Titanium mesh as an alternative to a membrane for ridge augmentation. *J. Oral Maxillofac. Surg.* **2012**, *70*, 803–810. [CrossRef]
26. Lizio, G.; Corinaldesi, G.; Marchetti, C. Alveolar ridge reconstruction with titanium mesh: A three-dimensional evaluation of factors affecting bone augmentation. *Int. J. Oral Maxillofac. Implant.* **2014**, 1354–1363. [CrossRef]
27. Poli, P.P.; Beretta, M.; Cicciù, M.; Maiorana, C. Alveolar ridge augmentation with titanium mesh. A retrospective clinical study. *Open Dent. J.* **2014**, *8*, 148–158. [CrossRef]

28. Sumida, T.; Otawa, N.; Kamata, Y.U.; Kamakura, S.; Mtsushita, T.; Kitagaki, H.; Mori, S.; Sasaki, K.; Fujibayashi, S.; Takemoto, M.; et al. Custom-made titanium devices as membranes for bone augmentation in implant treatment: Clinical application and the comparison with conventional titanium mesh. *J. Craniomaxillofac. Surg.* **2015**, *43*, 2183–2188.
29. Uehara, S.; Kurita, H.; Shimane, T.; Sakai, H.; Kamata, T.; Teramoto, Y.; Yamada, S. Predictability of staged localized alveolar ridge augmentation using a micro titanium mesh. *Oral Maxillofac. Surg.* **2015**, *19*, 411–416. [CrossRef]
30. Zita Gomes, R.; Paraud Freixas, A.; Han, C.H.; Bechara, S.; Tawil, I. Alveolar Ridge Reconstruction with Titanium Meshes and Simultaneous Implant Placement: A Retrospective, Multicenter Clinical Study. *Biomed. Res. Int.* **2016**, *2016*, 5126838. [CrossRef]
31. Andreasi Bassi, M.; Andrisani, C.; Lico, S.; Ormanier, Z.; Ottria, L.; Gargari, M. Guided bone regeneration via a preformed titanium foil: Clinical, histological and histomorphometric outcome of a case series. *Oral Implantol.* **2016**, *16*, 164–174.
32. Ciocca, L.; Lizio, G.; Baldissara, P.; Sambuco, A.; Scotti, R.; Corinaldesi, G. Prosthetically CAD-CAM-Guided Bone Augmentation of Atrophic Jaws Using Customized Titanium Mesh: Preliminary Results of an Open Prospective Study. *J. Oral Implantol.* **2018**, *44*, 131–137. [CrossRef]
33. Cucchi, A.; Sartori, M.; Parrilli, A.; Aldini, N.N.; Vignudelli, E.; Corinaldesi, G. Histological and histomorphometric analysis of bone tissue after guided bone regeneration with non-resorbable membranes vs. resorbable membranes and titanium mesh. *Clin. Implant. Dent. Relat. Res.* **2019**, *21*, 693–701. [CrossRef]
34. Zhang, T.; Zhang, T.; Cai, X. The application of a newly designed L-shaped titanium mesh for GBR with simultaneous implant placement in the esthetic zone: A retrospective case series study. *Clin. Implant. Dent. Relat. Res.* **2019**, *21*, 862–872. [CrossRef] [PubMed]
35. Atef, M.; Tarek, A.; Shaheen, M.; Alarawi, R.M.; Askar, N. Horizontal ridge augmentation using native collagen membrane vs. titanium mesh in atrophic maxillary ridges: Randomized clinical trial. *Clin. Implant. Dent. Relat. Res.* **2020**, *22*, 156–166. [CrossRef] [PubMed]
36. Malik, R.; Gupta, A.; Bansal, P.; Sharma, R.; Sharma, S. Evaluation of Alveolar Ridge Height Gained by Vertical Ridge Augmentation Using Titanium Mesh and Novabone Putty in Posterior Mandible. *J. Maxillofac. Oral Surg.* **2020**, *19*, 32–39. [CrossRef]
37. Cucchi, A.; Bianchi, A.; Calamai, P.; Rinaldi, L.; Mangano, F.; Vignudelli, E.; Corinaldesi, G. Clinical and volumetric outcomes after vertical ridge augmentation using computer-aided-design/computer-aided manufacturing (CAD/CAM) customized titanium meshes: A pilot study. *BMC Oral Health* **2020**, *20*, 219. [CrossRef] [PubMed]
38. Celletti, R.; Davarpanah, M.; Etienne, D.; Pecora, G.; Tecucianu, J.F.; Djukanovic, D.; Donath, K. Guided tissue regeneration around dental implants in immediate extraction sockets: Comparison of e-PTFE and a new titanium membrane. *Int. J. Periodontics Restor. Dent.* **1994**, *14*, 242–253.
39. Cucchi, A.; Vignudelli, E.; Napolitano, A.; Marchetti, C.; Corinaldesi, G. Evaluation of complication rates and vertical bone gain after guided bone regeneration with non-resorbable membranes versus titanium meshes and resorbable membranes. A randomized clinical trial. *Clin. Implant. Dent. Relat. Res.* **2017**, *19*, 821–832. [CrossRef] [PubMed]
40. Sagheb, K.; Schiegnitz, E.; Moergel, M.; Walter, C.; Al-Nawas, B.; Wagner, W. Clinical outcome of alveolar ridge augmentation with individualized CAD-CAM-produced titanium mesh. *Int. J. Implant. Dent.* **2017**, *3*, 36. [CrossRef] [PubMed]
41. Wessing, B.; Lettner, S.; Zechner, W. Guided Bone Regeneration with Collagen Membranes and Particulate Graft Materials: A Systematic Review and Meta-Analysis. *Int. J. Oral Maxillofac. Implant.* **2018**, *33*, 87–100. [CrossRef]
42. Roca-Millan, E.; Jané-Salas, E.; Estrugo-Devesa, A.; López-López, J. Evaluation of Bone Gain and Complication Rates after Guided Bone Regeneration with Titanium Foils: A Systematic Review. *Materials* **2020**, *13*, 5346. [CrossRef]
43. Lim, G.; Lin, G.H.; Monje, A.; Chan, H.L.; Wang, H.L. Wound Healing Complications Following Guided Bone Regeneration for Ridge Augmentation: A Systematic Review and Meta-Analysis. *Int. J. Oral Maxillofac. Implant.* **2018**, *33*, 41–50. [CrossRef] [PubMed]
44. Stenport, V.F.; Örtorp, A.; Thor, A. Onlay and inlay bone grafts with platelet-rich plasma: Histologic evaluations from human biopsies. *J. Oral Maxillofac. Surg.* **2011**, *69*, 1079–1085. [CrossRef] [PubMed]
45. Garcia, J.; Dodge, A.; Luepke, P.; Wang, H.L.; Kapila, Y.; Lin, G.H. Effect of membrane exposure on guided bone regeneration: A systematic review and meta-analysis. *Clin. Oral Implant. Res.* **2018**, *29*, 328–338. [CrossRef] [PubMed]
46. Benic, G.I.; Bernasconi, M.; Jung, R.E.; Hämmerle, C.H. Clinical and radiographic intra-subject comparison of implants placed with or without guided bone regeneration: 15-year results. *J. Clin. Periodontol.* **2017**, *44*, 315–325. [CrossRef]
47. Clementini, M.; Morlupi, A.; Canullo, L.; Agrestini, C.; Barlattani, A. Success rate of dental implants inserted in horizontal and vertical guided bone regenerated areas: A systematic review. *Int. J. Oral Maxillofac. Surg.* **2012**, *41*, 847–855. [CrossRef] [PubMed]

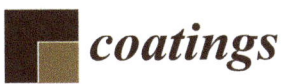

Article

Highly Bioactive Elastomeric Hybrid Nanoceramics for Guiding Bone Tissue Regeneration

Jing Chen [1,2,*], Wenxiu Que [2,*], Bo Lei [3] and Beibei Li [1]

1. The Key Laboratory for Surface Engineering and Remanufacturing in Shaanxi Province, School of Chemical Engineering, Xi'an University, Xi'an 710065, China
2. Electronic Materials Research Laboratory, International Center for Dielectric Research, Key Laboratory of the Ministry of Education, School of Electronic & Information Engineering, Xi'an Jiaotong University, Xi'an 710054, China
3. Frontier Institute of Science and Technology, Xi'an Jiaotong University, Xi'an 710054, China

* Correspondence: jingchen@xawl.edu.cn (J.C.); wxque@mail.xjtu.edu.cn (W.Q.); Tel./Fax: +86-29-83385679 (W.Q.)

Abstract: Conventional bioactive ceramic implants possess high osteogenic ability but exhibit poor machinability and brittleness, which limit their wide applications. In this study, we report an elastomeric machinable bioactive nanoceramic-based hybrid membrane that is formed by nanohydroxyapatite-reinforced hybrid matrix (poly(dimethylsilicone)-bioactive glass-poly(caprolactone) (nHA-PBP)) using a modified sol-gel process. The hybrid matrix is composed of elastomeric polydimethylsiloxane and bioactive glass nanogel. The effect of the nHA contents (0, 20, 30, 40 and 50 wt%) on the physicochemical structure and biomineralization activity of PBP hybrid membranes is investigated systematically. The results show that nHA-PBP hybrid membranes containing more than 20 wt% nHA exhibit the highest apatite-forming bioactivity due to the optimized hydroxyapatite crystalline phase. NHA-PBP implants with nHA also show good elastomeric mechanical behavior and foldable mechanical properties. Furthermore, the study of the in vitro cellular biocompatibility suggests that the nHA-PBP hybrid monoliths can enhance osteoblast (MC3T3-E1) attachment and proliferation. The biomimetic hybrid composition, crack-free monolith structure, and high biological activity of apatite formation make the nHA-PBP hybrid membrane a prospective candidate in the application of bone tissue regeneration.

Keywords: bioactive materials; bioactive ceramic; bioactive glass; nanohydroxyapatite; sol-gel process

Citation: Chen, J.; Que, W.; Lei, B.; Li, B. Highly Bioactive Elastomeric Hybrid Nanoceramics for Guiding Bone Tissue Regeneration. *Coatings* **2022**, *12*, 1633. https://doi.org/10.3390/coatings12111633

Academic Editor: Jun-Beom Park

Received: 5 October 2022
Accepted: 25 October 2022
Published: 27 October 2022

Publisher's Note: MDPI stays neutral with regard to jurisdictional claims in published maps and institutional affiliations.

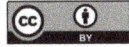

Copyright: © 2022 by the authors. Licensee MDPI, Basel, Switzerland. This article is an open access article distributed under the terms and conditions of the Creative Commons Attribution (CC BY) license (https://creativecommons.org/licenses/by/4.0/).

1. Introduction

Bioactive glass-based biomaterials (BGs) have shown successful applications in bone tissue repair and regeneration due to their good biocompatibility, osteoconductivity, and bone-bonding ability when implanted in vivo without any interfaces of fibrous connective tissue [1–4]. This high bone-bonding ability with living bone tissue is considered to be highly associated with their bone-like apatite layer formation [5]. Because BG has a high conductivity and bone bondability, and enhanced bone regeneration potential, the application of BG-based biomaterials in bone tissue regeneration has widely attracted attention in recent years [6]. However, pure BG is limited for use in bone tissue engineering applications due to its inherent brittleness and low flexibility. Furthermore, it is difficult for BG to form various shapes for improving in vivo applications. Hence, there is a considerable need to design and fabricate highly bioactive glass-based biomaterials with tough mechanical properties for bone tissue engineering applications.

As compared with inorganic bioactive glass materials, biopolymers exhibit unique biological physical and biochemical properties, such as high toughness, electrometric properties, greater capacity for body fluid absorption, and better gel forming capacity [7]. Hence, it is reasonable to incorporate inorganic nanoparticles into a polymer matrix to produce nanocomposites with optimized physicochemical properties, such as bioactive glass micro-nanoscale particles-poly(caprolactone) (MNBG-PCL) biomaterials [8,9]. Actually, the addition of bioactive phases significantly improves the mechanical modulus, biomineralization activity, and biocompatibility in osteoblasts of the PCL matrix [10–12], but a particle-based inorganic phase is an obstacle to the enhancement of the strength and toughness of the polymer simultaneously due to its poor interactions [13]. Recently, molecular-level-based silica-based glass sol was added into a polymer solution to synthesize the bioactive glass–polymer hybrid biomaterials, including BG-PCL, BG-gelatin, BG-chitosan, and BG-poly(ethylene glycol) [14–16]. In the case of the molecular hybridization, the obtained hybrids show the stable mechanical property, biomineralization activity, and osteoblast biocompatibility. As a result, the development of silica-based hybrid polymer biomaterials for effective bone tissue regeneration applications is highly promising [17].

In the guiding bone tissue regeneration application, the guiding membrane biomaterials are crucial to enhance the tissue repair through preventing the invasion of external protein and cells [18]. The ideal guiding membrane should be tough, bioactive, and easy-handling. In our previous work, poly(dimethylsilicone)-bioactive glass-PCL (PBP) hybrid membranes without fracture were successfully fabricated via a sol-gel process, which exhibited a controlled surface morphology, mechanical property, and biomineralization [10]. There is still much space to improve the apatite-forming ability (biomineralization activity) and osteoblast biocompatibility of the PBP hybrid membrane. Human bone tissue is a typical organic–inorganic composite consisting of nano-crystalline hydroxyapatite (nHA) and collagen polymer. Artificial HA has received more attention as a bioactive ceramic material in bone replacement and repair applications due to its similar structure and composition to natural apatite. It was selected as an inorganic additive for biomimicking. In addition, some published works suggest that HA supplementation can provide pH buffers for acid-released production [19–21]. In this regard, incorporating nanoscale HA into biomaterials may be a promising option for enhancing biomineralization activity and osteoblastic ability.

In this study, the crack-free nHA-PBP hybrid membranes are prepared via a typical sol-gel method. The effects of the addition of nanoscale HA (nHA) on the structural property and biomineralization activity of the PBP hybrids are also investigated. In addition, the purpose of this study is to analyze the effects of nHA-PBP hybrid membranes with different HA loading concentrations on cell attachment to examine the basic biocompatibility of hybrid materials. It is anticipated that the incorporation of nHA can significantly improve the biomineralization and osteoblastic biocompatibility of the nHA-PBP hybrid biomaterials.

2. Experimental

2.1. Materials

Tetraethoxysilane (TEOS, $Si(OC_2H_5)_4$), calcium nitrite ($Ca(NO_3)_2 \cdot 4H_2O$), isopropyl-alcohol (IPA), tetrahydrofuran (THF), dichloromethane (DCM), and hydrochloric acid (HCl, 35%) were obtained from Guanghua Chemical Factory Co., Ltd. (Guangzhou, China). Polydimethylsiloxane (PDMS, HO-[$Si(CH_3)_2$-O-]$_n$H, Mn = 1100) was provided by Alfa (Alfa, Ward Hill, MA, USA). Poly(caprolactone) (PCL, $(C_6H_{10}O_2)_n$) (M_n = 80,000) was supplied by Sigma-Aldrich (Sigma-Aldrich, St. Louis, MO, USA). Nano-hydroxyapatite (nHA) powder (consisting of loose aggregates of approximately 100 nm crystals) was purchased from Alfa Aesar (Ward Hill, MA, USA)

2.2. Synthesis of nHA-PBP Hybrid Membrane

The nHA-PBP hybrid membranes were synthesized. Briefly, 10 mL IPA and 20 mL THF were combined to form co-blended solvents, TEOS (6.5 g) was first dissolved in this aqueous solution. Thirty minutes later, 1.5 mL of 35% HCL, 12 mL of water, and 2.2 g of PDMS were added into the solution for completely catalyzation and hydrolyzed reaction for 30 min. Then, the $Ca(NO_3)_2 \cdot 4H_2O$, IPA, and H_2O were added to the aforementioned solution. The generated bioactive PDMS-BG sol was then mixed with the DCM solution of PCL and further stirred for 30 min. To obtain the nHA-PBP hybrid sol, the predetermined containing nHA (0, 20, 30, 40, and 50 wt% relative to the PCL polymer) was added and vigorously stirred for 20 h. Then, the mixture was poured into the Teflon dishes and dried at 37 °C for 12 h to form the nHA-PBP mixed gel. Finally, after heating the mixed gel at 60 °C for 12 h, the nHA-PBP hybrid membranes were obtained.

2.3. Characterization of the Specimens

Scanning electron microscopy (SEM, JSM-6390, JEOL, Tokyo, Japan) was used to characterize the surface microstructural and morphological properties of samples. The elemental composition of the samples was evaluated by energy dispersive spectrometry (EDS, JEOL, Tokyo, Japan). The crystalline phase structure of the hybrid membranes were studied through Cu Kα radiation measured by X-ray diffraction of radiation, performed at 40 kV and 30 mA; the scanning speed was 0.02°/s and the step size was 0.02°, ranging from 15° to 60° (XRD, D/MAX-2400, Rigaku, Tokyo, Japan).

2.4. Mechanical Behavior Assessment of Hybrids

The universal mechanical devices (SHT4206, MTS, Minneapolis, MN, USA) with a 500 N load cell was used to evaluate the tensile mechanical characteristics (tensile strength and modulus) of hybrid monoliths at a crosshead speed of 50 mm per minute. All samples with a size of 10 mm × 60 mm were used for the tensile mechanical test. The stress–strain curves were captured by the additional software of the machine. The tensile modulus of samples was obtained by determining the slope of the initial linear elastic portion of stress–strain curves. At least five species were counted in each sample.

2.5. Biomineralization Activity

According to our previous report, the specimens incubated in simulated body fluid (SBF) for a certain time to determine the biomineralization activity of hybrid membranes [22]. After soaking, the formation of apatite on the surface of the sample was tested. Briefly, the samples were cut into a size of $10 \times 10 \times 2$ mm^3 and incubated in SBF with a similar composition to human blood plasma (in mM: Ca^{2+} 2.5, Mg^{2+} 1.5, Na^+ 142, K^+ 5.0, SO_4^{2-} 0.5, HPO_4^{2-} 1.0, Cl^- 147.8, HCO_3^- 4.2). After 7 days of incubation at 37 °C, the samples were taken out of the fluids and washed with deionized water to remove the specimen. Then, the samples were dried at 40 °C for 24 h. Then, the activity of apatite forming on the surface of the samples was analyzed by SEM, EDS, and XRD.

2.6. Cell Proliferation and Viability of the Hybrid Membranes

The cellular biocompatibility of the hybrid membrane was evaluated by using the osteoblast cell line (MC3T3-E1). Cells were cultured in a standard Dulbecco's modified essential medium (DMEM, Invitrogen) in a humidified atmosphere with 5% CO_2 and supplemented with 10% fetal calf serum (FCS). All samples with a size of 10 mm × 10 mm were sterilized by ultraviolet (UV) irradiation for 30 min on each side before cell seeding. MC3T3-E1 cells were seeded on the surface of the hybrid materials at a density of 5000 cells per well. The cell attachment and morphology were then evaluated with a LIVE/DEAD viability kit (Molecular Probes) after the 3-day culture. The staining procedure was according to the manufacture instruction. The cell morphology was observed with a fluorescence microscope (IX53, Olympus, Tokyo, Japan).

After the incubation for 1, 3, and 5 days, the cell viability and proliferation were determined by using a commercial Alamar Blue™ assay kit (Life Technologies). A tissue culture plate (TCP) was used as a control. The cell metabolic activity after incubation with an Alamar Blue kit was performed by a microplate reader (Molecular Devices) according to the instruction book. At least 5 species per sample were analyzed to obtain mean value and standard deviation (SD).

2.7. Statistics Analysis

Mean ± standard deviation (SD) indicated all data. The student's test analysis of Social Science Statistical Program Software (SPSS 19.0, Inc., Chicago, IL, USA) used to detect the statistical differences between the groups of measurements. Statistically significant difference was represented as * p less than 0.05 and ** p less than 0.01.

3. Results and Discussion

3.1. Morphological Measurement

Through the direct hybridization of PDMS-BG sol, PCL solution, and nHA, the nHA-PBP hybrids were successfully obtained as shown in Figure 1. After thermal casting and incubation, the crack-free hybrid membrane formed. In the hybrid structure, PDMS may have a strong interaction with BG sol through the Si-O-Si bonds. Furthermore, the hydrophobic alkyl chains may have high affinity with the PCL phase. Therefore, the molecular-level inorganic–organic phase structure of the as-fabricated hybrid membranes can be facilely formed. In addition, the nanoscale HA particles are efficiently incorporated into the PBP matrix, which may enhance their surface nanostructure and bioactivity, as well as the osteoblasts biocompatibility.

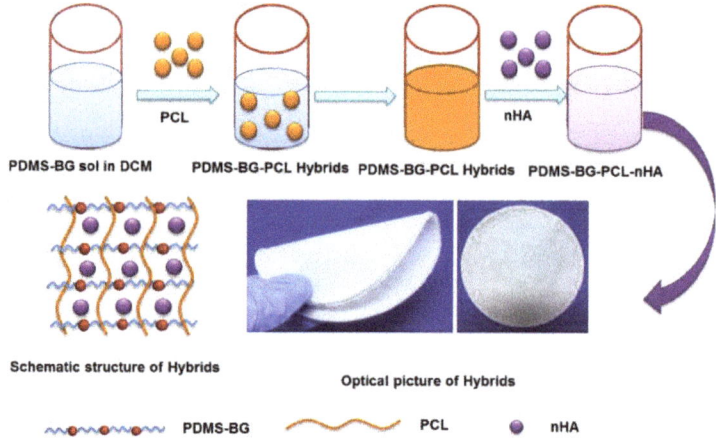

Figure 1. Process diagram and optical images of crack-free nHA-PBP hybrid monoliths fabricated by the representative sol-gel route.

Figure 2 reveals the crystalline phase composition and structure of the as-fabricated nHA-PBP hybrids with various amounts of nHA (0, 20, 30, 40, and 50 wt%) by XRD characterization. In spite of the variations observed in crystallization, one can clearly observe the XRD peaks at $2\theta = 21.88°$ and $2\theta = 23.85°$, which are ascribed to the representative characteristic peaks of the PCL (semi-crystalline polymer). It is also observed that the PCL peaks significantly decrease in intensity with the increase in nHA content (20–50 wt%). Furthermore, the appearance and significant enhancement in intensity of the peaks at 32°, 46°, and 49° demonstrates the presence of nHA in the nHA-PBP hybrids.

The surface microstructures and morphologies of the nHA-PBP hybrid membranes containing different nHA contents are shown in Figure 3. It can be observed that the surface roughness of the hybrids increases significantly with the addition of nHA. There are some joints and protuberances on the surface of these composites, which indicates that HA nanoparticles are attached to PCL surfaces. The SEM images also show that the HA particles (particle areas) density increases when the loading concentration increases (Figure 3C–E). Figure 4 shows EDS spectra of the nHA-PBP hybrid membranes. The results confirm that calcium (Ca), phosphorous (P), carbon (C), and oxygen (O) are present in the matrix. The diagram demonstrates that the chemical composition changes with the addition of different nHA contents. The Ca and P peaks in intensity significantly rise with the increase in nHA content. These results reveal that nHA can be effectively crosslinked and hybridized with the PBP matrix.

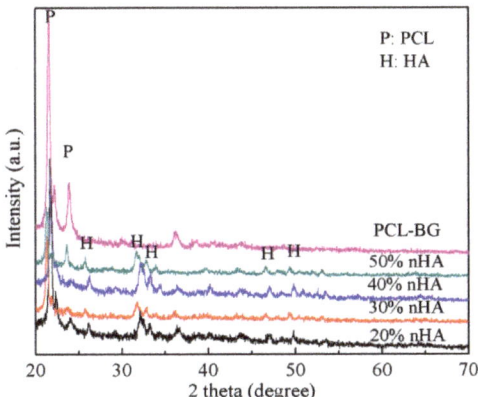

Figure 2. XRD patterns of the nHA-PBP hybrid membranes with different nHA contents.

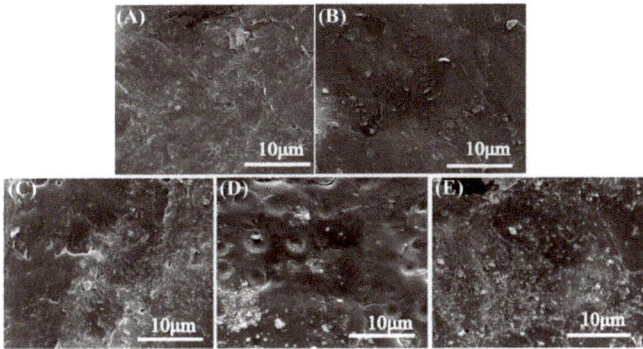

Figure 3. Surface microstructures and morphologies of the nHA-PBP hybrid membranes. (**A**) 0 wt% nHA, (**B**) 20 wt% nHA, (**C**) 30 wt% nHA, (**D**) 40 wt% nHA, (**E**) 50 wt% nHA.

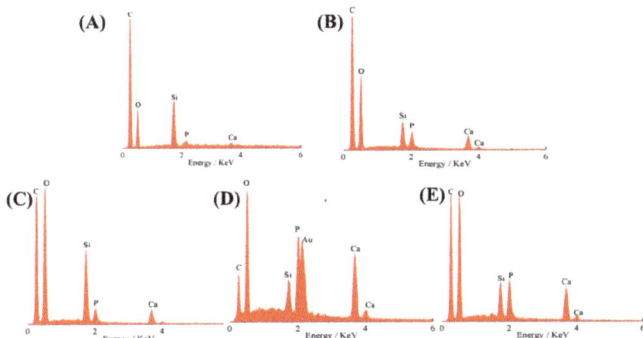

Figure 4. EDS analysis spectra of the nHA-PBP hybrid membranes. (**A**) 0 wt% nHA, (**B**) 20 wt% nHA, (**C**) 30 wt% nHA, (**D**) 40 wt% nHA, (**E**) 50 wt% nHA.

3.2. Mechanical Properties Assessment of the nHA-PBP Hybrid Membranes

The tensile tests are used to assess the mechanical properties of nHA-PBP hybrid membranes, as shown in Figure 5. Figure 5A shows the tensile stress–strain behavior of nHA-PBP hybrids with varying nHA contents (20, 30, 40 wt%). All samples show representative stress–strain behaviors in the initial 10% stain range. The ultimate tensile strength of hybrid membranes decreased from 4.77 ± 0.30 to 2.77 ± 0.25 MPa with increasing nHA content from 20 to 40 wt% (Figure 5B). The Young's modulus of nHA-PBP 20 wt% hybrids indicated a high value of 87.94 ± 1.32 MPa as compared to the 59.58 ± 2.54 of 40 wt% (Figure 5C). The failure stress showed a similar tendency to change with ultimate tensile strength for nHA-PBP from 20 to 40 wt% (Figure 5D). The results show that increasing the amount of nHA in the nHA-PBP hybrids reduced flexural strength. When the nHA content is high, the nHA may not be hybridized well with the polymer phase, and the uniform structure may induce the decrease in flexural strength. Since nHA has poor mechanical properties, its utilization is limited to clinical load bearing applications. To make nHA-PBP hybrid materials play an important role in bone regeneration, some weaknesses of each component need to be improved in order to provide excellent quality and interfacial attachment of new bone tissue.

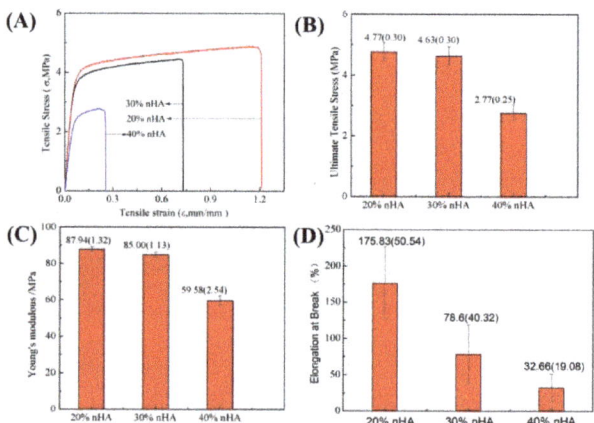

Figure 5. Mechanical properties assessment of nHA-PBP hybrid membranes with different nHA contents. (**A**) Stress–strain behavior; (**B**) Ultimate tensile strength; (**C**) Young's modulus; (**D**) Elongation at break.

3.3. Biomineralization Activity of the nHA-PBP Hybrid Membranes

Considering that the biomineralization activity critically influences the biomaterials in bone tissue regeneration, here, the bioactivity of the nHA-PBP hybrid membranes for in vitro apatite forming is assessed by immersion in SBF for 7 days. As shown in Figure 6, the apatite formation capability of the hybrid membranes is significantly affected by the nHA contents. As one can see in Figure 6, the surface of the nHA-PBP hybrid membranes shows new apatite layers relative to the specimens before incubation in SBF (in Figure 3). That is, the mineral is deposited and aggregated in the form of a globular accumulation on the surface of the sample with 0 wt% nHA of the nHA-PBP hybrid membranes as in Figure 6A,B. When the additive of nHA increases to 20 wt% and 30 wt%, the nHA-PBP is covered with densely spherically shaped particles as seen in Figure 6C–F. With the nHA content increasing, the surface morphology of the as-formed hydroxyapatite nanocrystals changes considerably. In addition, it progressively shows needle-like or rod-like characteristics in shape, as shown in Figure 6H,J, showing typical biomineralization characteristics only for bioactive glass materials.

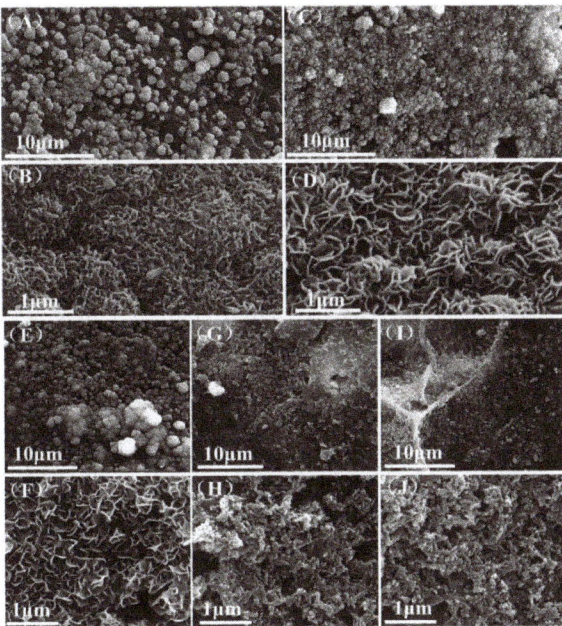

Figure 6. Surface morphologies of the nHA-PBP hybrid membranes with different nHA contents after biomineralization in SBF for 7 days. (**A,B**) 0 wt% nHA, (**C,D**) 20 wt% nHA, (**E,F**) 30 wt% nHA, (**G,H**) 40 wt% nHA, (**I,J**) 50 wt% nHA.

Figure 7 shows the EDS spectra of the nHA-PBP hybrid membranes with various nHA contents after being immersed into SBF for 7 days. It can be seen that, compared to the EDS of the hybrid membrane before being soaked, immersion into SBF leads to the formation of the hydroxyapatite. As the nHA content increases, the formation of hydroxyapatite increases, which is accordant with the published literature. In addition, EDS of the hybrid membrane with the addition of 20 wt% nHA, after being soaked in SBF, shows a significant decrease in the calcium content, indicating a biological apatite formation with a calcium-deficient characteristic [23].

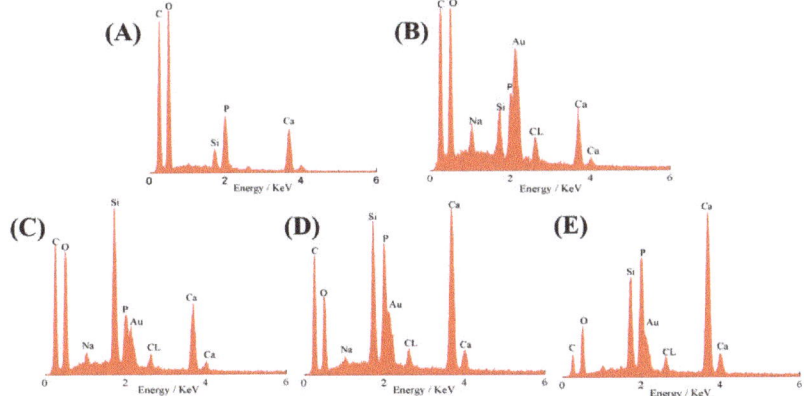

Figure 7. Elemental compositions of the nHA-PBP hybrid membranes with different nHA contents after biomineralization in SBF for 7 days. (**A**) 0 wt% (**B**) 20 wt%; (**C**) 30 wt%; (**D**) 40 wt%; (**E**) 50 wt%.

Figure 8 shows the XRD patterns of the hybrid membranes containing different nHA contents and after the 7 days of incubation in SBF, which are employed to investigate the structure of the crystalline phase property of the new forming apatite layer on the hybrid membrane surface. These results indicate that several characteristic peaks are related to crystalline hydroxyapatite. It is also clear to see that the peaks referring to PCL at 2θ = 21.88° and 2θ = 23.85° are significantly weakened in intensity after 7 days of soaking in SBF, which implies the newly mineralized apatite layer forming on the specimens film. The XRD diffraction peaks at 32°, 39°, 46°, and 49° for the hybrids with the addition of 20–50 wt% of nHA correspond to the crystal planes of (211), (310), (222), and (213) of the HA (JCPDS No. 09-0432) [21]. It should be noted that the characteristic peaks of HA are not obvious for the pure PBP hybrid. Clearly, these SEM, EDS, and XRD results demonstrate that the nHA incorporation can remarkably increase the capability for biomineralization in the nHA-PBP hybrid membranes.

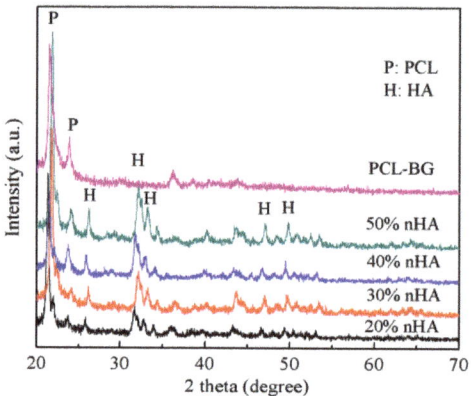

Figure 8. XRD patterns of the nHA-PBP hybrid membranes with different nHA contents after biomineralization in SBF for 7 days. Representative diffraction peaks of hydroxyapatite were marked in the patterns.

3.4. Osteoblasts Biocompatibility Assessment of the nHA-PBP Hybrid Membranes

Figure 9 shows the cell attachment and proliferation activity of the osteoblast line (MC3T3-E1) after culturing for 1, 3, and 5 days on the surface of the hybrid membranes. The cells show normal attachment and spreading morphology on the surface of the PBP hybrid membrane, as shown in Figure 9A. While for the nHA-PBP 20 wt% (in Figure 9B) and the nHA-PBP 50 wt% (in Figure 9C) after being cultured for 5 days, there are no significant dead cells observed on the surface of these samples, demonstrating their good cell attachment ability. There are high cell numbers on the surfaces of the hybrid membrane with the incorporation of 20 wt% and 50 wt% nHA compared to the pure PBP hybrid membrane, further suggesting their enhanced cellular biocompatibility. In addition, the cell viability on the PCL and the nHA-PBP hybrid membranes significantly increases as the culture period extends from 1 day to 5 days, which indicates that the as-fabricated hybrid membranes can support the osteoblast proliferation, as seen in Figure 9D. Compared to the PBP control, the osteoblast presents significantly high cell viability after incubating with the nHA-PBP (20% and 50%) for 5 day culture periods. The cell viability is significantly improved as the nHA incorporation increases. These results demonstrate that our nHA-PBP hybrid membranes possess a good osteoblast biocompatibility and the incorporation of nHA can efficiently improve the osteoblast activity of the PBP hybrid membranes.

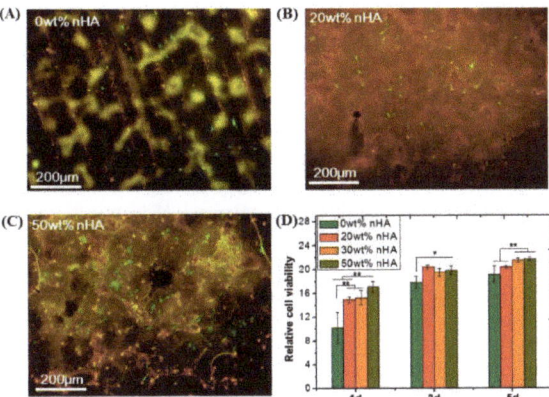

Figure 9. Osteoblasts biocompatibility investigation of the nHA-PBP hybrid membranes with different nHA contents (20 wt% and 50 wt% nHA). MC3T3-E1 cell attachment morphology at 3 days ((**A**), 0 wt%, (**B**), 20 wt% and (**C**), 50 wt% nHA) and proliferation activity after 1–5 days of culture (**D**). * $p < 0.05$ and ** $p < 0.01$ represent the significance differences between groups (n = 5).

In our previous work, the crack-free PBP hybrid membrane was successfully prepared by a conventional sol-gel method, which developed the functional hybrid membranes by incorporating HA particles into PBP sol. The relation between the hybrid properties and apatite-forming bioactivity was investigated, as well as attachment and proliferation in vitro. As one knows, PDMS is well compatible with silicon-based sol phase because it has a typical Si-O-Si skeleton chain and side chain, which induces a strong interaction with the hydrophobic PCL polymer. However, the biomineralization capability and biocompatibility of osteoblasts with the materials still need further improvement. Due to its highly biomimetic chemical structure and composition, HA is a typical bioactive ceramic and was successfully used in bone regeneration. The SEM results show that the HA particles can be uniformly dispersed into the PCL matrix. As a result, in this material system, it is easy to form a homogeneous inorganic–organic hybrid structure. The additive of nHA significantly enhances the biomineralization activity (apatite-forming ability) of the PBP hybrid membranes, as previously reported [24–26]. It is known that MC3T3-E1 cells have different reactions to changes in hybrid surface properties. The surface roughness of these two samples (i.e., 0 wt% and 20 wt% of the nHA) was not significantly different (Figure 3A,B), the number of attached cells on nHA 20 wt% was slightly higher than that of the nHA 0 wt%. This suggests that MC3T3-E1 cells prefer HA-containing samples to adhesion and proliferation. One possible explanation is that HA exists on a composite surface, resulting in more permanent interaction with adsorbed protein. It is absorbed by serums and proteins in the culture medium, or the protein is absorbed by the cell itself. It is also apparent that the cells are distributed more evenly on the nHA-PBP hybrid membrane surface (Figure 9B,C), which further suggests that HA favors the uniform distribution of adsorbed proteins. The addition of nHA also greatly enhances the osteoblasts biocompatibility of the as-fabricated PBP hybrid membranes. In addition, these results match earlier studies that reported the important role of nHA in polymer nanocomposites [27–29].

In bone tissue regeneration applications, the ideal biomaterials should be facilely synthesized and have high bioactivities, including biomineralization activity, for bone-bonding and osteoblast biocompatibility for regeneration. However, the PBP hybrid membrane needs a long processing time (more than 72 h), which is unfavorable for large-scale production and, thereby, limits applications. Based on the requirement for reducing the processing time and enhancing biomineralization activity and osteoblast biocompatibility, the present new developed nHA-PBP hybrid membranes may have promising applications in future bone tissue regeneration.

4. Conclusions

To sum up, highly bioactive and crack-free nHA-PBP hybrid membrane ingredients were successfully prepared via the conventional sol-gel method. Results indicate that adding HA can significantly improve the surface roughness and biomineralization activity of hybrid membranes. The nHA-PBP hybrid membranes after being soaked in SBF can easily induce a crystalline apatite layer on the surface, indicating their excellent biomineralization activity. The optimized nHA-PBP hybrids also show significantly enhanced osteoblast biocompatibility. The hybrids containing 20 wt% nHA show an optimized elastic modulus and toughness. The crack-free structure, short processing time, and high bioactivity of the production of hydroxyapatite formation and biomimetic hybrid composition make the as-fabricated nHA-PBP hybrid membrane a desired candidate as a guidance membrane for future applications in biomedical materials.

Author Contributions: Methodology, J.C. and B.L. (Bo Lei).; software, J.C. and B.L. (Beibei Li); investigation, J.C.; writing—original draft preparation, J.C.; writing—review and editing, J.C., B.L. (Bo Lei) and W.Q.; funding acquisition, J.C. and B.L. (Beibei Li). All authors have read and agreed to the published version of the manuscript.

Funding: This research was funded by the Natural Science Basic Research Plan in Shaanxi Province of China (No. 2019JM-520 and 2020JQ-890), the 3-year action plan of Xi'an University (2021xdjh34).

Institutional Review Board Statement: Not applicable.

Informed Consent Statement: Not applicable.

Data Availability Statement: All the data supporting the results of the study are included in the paper.

Conflicts of Interest: The authors declare no conflict of interest.

References

1. Kaur, G.; Kumar, V.; Baino, F.; Mauro, J.C.; Pickrell, G.; Evans, L.; Bretcanu, O. Mechanical properties of bioactive glasses, ceramics, glass-ceramics and composites: State-of-the-art review and future challenges. *Mater. Sci. Eng. C* **2019**, *104*, 109895.
2. Hum, J.; Boccaccini, A.R. Bioactive glasses as carriers for bioactive molecules and therapeutic drugs: A review. *J. Mater. Sci. Mater. Med.* **2012**, *23*, 2317–2333. [CrossRef]
3. Furlan, R.G.; Correr, W.R.; Russi, A.F.C.; da Costa Iemma, M.R.; Trovatti, E.; Pecoraro, É. Preparation and characterization of boron-based bioglass by sol–gel process. *J. Sol-Gel Sci. Technol.* **2018**, *88*, 181–191. [CrossRef]
4. Kaur, G.; Pandey, O.P.; Singh, K.; Homa, D.; Scott, B.; Pickrell, G. A review of bioactive glasses: Their structure, properties, fabrication and apatite formation. *J. Biomed. Mater. Res. A* **2014**, *102*, 254–274. [CrossRef] [PubMed]
5. Biswal, T. Biopolymers for tissue engineering applications: A review. *Mater. Today* **2021**, *41*, 397–402. [CrossRef]
6. Lei, B.; Guo, B.; Rambhia, K.J.; Ma, P.X. Hybrid polymer biomaterials for bone tissue regeneration. *Front. Med.* **2019**, *13*, 189–201. [CrossRef]
7. Ozdil, D.; Murat Aydin, H. Polymers for medical and tissue engineering applications. *J. Chem. Technol. Biotechnol.* **2014**, *89*, 1793–1810. [CrossRef]
8. Chen, J.; Que, W.; Xing, Y.; Lei, B. Molecular level-based bioactive glass-poly (caprolactone) hybrids monoliths with porous structure for bone tissue repair. *Ceram. Int.* **2015**, *41*, 3330–3334. [CrossRef]
9. Lei, B.; Shin, K.H.; Noh, D.Y.; Jo, I.H.; Koh, Y.H.; Kim, H.E.; Kim, S.E. Sol–gel derived nanoscale bioactive glass (NBG) particles reinforced poly (ε-caprolactone) composites for bone tissue engineering. *Mater. Sci. Eng. C* **2013**, *33*, 1102–1108. [CrossRef]
10. Chen, J.; Du, Y.; Que, W.; Xing, Y.; Lei, B. Content-dependent biomineralization activity and mechanical properties based on polydimethylsiloxane–bioactive glass–poly(caprolactone) hybrids monoliths for bone tissue regeneration. *RSC Adv.* **2015**, *5*, 61309–61317. [CrossRef]
11. Pires, L.S.O.; Fernandes, M.H.F.V.; de Oliveira, J.M.M. Crystallization kinetics of PCL and PCL–glass composites for additive manufacturing. *J. Therm. Anal. Calorim.* **2018**, *134*, 2115–2125. [CrossRef]
12. Mohammadkhah, A.; Marquardt, L.M.; Sakiyama-Elbert, S.E.; Day, D.E.; Harkins, A.B. Fabrication and characterization of poly-(ε)-caprolactone and bioactive glass composites for tissue engineering applications. *Mater. Sci. Eng. C* **2015**, *49*, 632–639. [CrossRef] [PubMed]
13. Ma, J.; Wu, C. Bioactive inorganic particles-based biomaterials for skin tissue engineering. *Exploration* **2022**, *2*, 20210083. [CrossRef]
14. Sohrabi, M.; Eftekhari Yekta, B.; Rezaie, H.; Naimi-Jamal, M.R.; Kumar, A.; Cochis, A.; Miola, M.; Rimondini, L. Enhancing Mechanical Properties and Biological Performances of Injectable Bioactive Glass by Gelatin and Chitosan for Bone Small Defect Repair. *Biomedicine* **2020**, *8*, 616. [CrossRef] [PubMed]

15. Erol-Taygun, M.; Unalan, I.; Idris, M.I.B.; Mano, J.F.; Boccaccini, A.R. Bioactive Glass-Polymer Nanocomposites for Bone Tissue Regeneration Applications: A Review. *Adv. Eng. Mater.* **2019**, *21*, 1900287. [CrossRef]
16. Chen, J.; Que, W.; Xing, Y.; Lei, B. Highly bioactive polysiloxane modified bioactive glass-poly (ethylene glycol) hybrids monoliths with controlled surface structure for bone tissue regeneration. *Appl. Surf. Sci.* **2015**, *332*, 542–548. [CrossRef]
17. Wu, W.; Wang, W.; Li, J. Star polymers: Advances in biomedical applications. *Progress Polym. Sci.* **2015**, *46*, 55–85. [CrossRef]
18. Gao, W.; Xiao, Y. Advances in cell membrane-encapsulated biomaterials for tissue repair and regeneration. *Appl. Mater. Today* **2022**, *26*, 101389. [CrossRef]
19. Tavakol, S.; Azami, M.; Khoshzaban, A.; Ragerdi Kashani, I.; Tavakol, B.; Hoveizi, E.; Rezayat Sorkhabadi, S.M. Effect of laminated hydroxyapatite/gelatin nanocomposite scaffold structure on osteogenesis using unrestricted somatic stem cells in rat. *Cell Biol. Int.* **2013**, *37*, 1181–1189. [CrossRef]
20. Kim, H.W.; Kim, H.E.; Salih, V. Stimulation of Osteoblast Responses to Biomimetic Nanocomposites of Gelatin-Hydroxyapatite for Tissue Engineering Scaffolds. *Biomaterials* **2005**, *26*, 5221–5230. [CrossRef]
21. Sadeghi-Avalshahr, A.; Khorsand-Ghayeni, M.; Nokhasteh, S.; Mahdavi Shahri, M.; Molavi, A.M.; Sadeghi-Avalshahr, M. Effects of hydroxyapatite (HA) particles on the PLLA polymeric matrix for fabrication of absorbable interference screws. *Polym. Bull.* **2018**, *75*, 2559–2574. [CrossRef]
22. Chen, J.; Que, W.; He, Z.; Zhang, X. PDMS-modified CaO-SiO$_2$ hybrids derived by a sol–gel process for biomedical applications. *Polym. Compos.* **2014**, *35*, 1193–1197. [CrossRef]
23. Hutchens, S.A.; Benson, R.S.; Evans, B.R.; O'Neill, H.M.; Rawn, C.J. Biomimetic synthesis of calcium-deficient hydroxyapatite in a natural hydrogel. *Biomaterials* **2006**, *27*, 4661–4670. [CrossRef]
24. Zhang, Y.; Reddy, V.J.; Wong, S.Y.; Li, X.; Su, B.; Ramakrishna, S.; Lim, C.T. Enhanced biomineralization in osteoblasts on a novel electrospun biocomposite nanofibrous substrate of hydroxyapatite/collagen/chitosan. *Tissue Eng. Part A* **2010**, *16*, 1949–1960. [CrossRef]
25. Altamura, D.; Pastore, S.G.; Raucci, M.G.; Siliqi, D.; De Pascalis, F.; Nacucchi, M.; Ambrosio, L.; Giannini, C. Scanning Small- and Wide-Angle X-ray Scattering Microscopy Selectively Probes HA Content in Gelatin/Hydroxyapatite Scaffolds for Osteochondral Defect Repair. *ACS Appl. Mater. Interfaces* **2016**, *8*, 8728–8736. [CrossRef]
26. Li, M.; Liu, W.; Sun, J.; Xianyu, Y.; Wang, J.; Zhang, W.; Zheng, W.; Huang, D.; Di, S.; Long, Y.-Z. Jiang, X. Culturing Primary Human Osteoblasts on Electrospun Poly (lactic-co-glycolic acid) and Poly (lactic-co-glycolic acid)/Nanohydroxy apatite Scaffolds for Bone Tissue Engineering. *ACS Appl. Mater. Interfaces* **2013**, *5*, 5921–5926. [CrossRef] [PubMed]
27. Perssona, M.; Loritea, G.S.; Kokkonena, H.E.; Choc, S.W.; Lehenkari, P.P.; Skrifvars, M.; Tuukkanena, J. Effect of bioactive extruded PLA/HA composite films on focal adhesion formation of preosteoblastic cells. *Colloids Surf. B* **2014**, *121*, 409–416. [CrossRef] [PubMed]
28. Kobayashi, M.; Nihonmatsu, S.; Okawara, T.; Onuki, H.; Sakagami, H.; Nakajima, H.; Takeishi, H.; Shimada, J. Adhesion and Proliferation of Osteoblastic Cells on Hydroxyapatite-dispersed Ti-based Composite Plate. *In Vivo* **2019**, *33*, 1067–1079. [CrossRef]
29. Monmaturapoj, N.; Srion, A.; Chalermkarnon, P.; Buchatip, S.; Petchsuk, A.; Noppakunmongkolchai, W.; Mai-Ngam, K. Properties of poly (lactic acid)/hydroxyapatite composite through the use of epoxy functional compatibilizers for biomedical application. *J. Biomater. Appl.* **2017**, *32*, 088532821771578. [CrossRef]

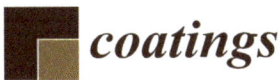

Article

Evaluation of *Streptococcus mutans* Adhesion to Stainless Steel Surfaces Modified Using Different Topographies Following a Biomimetic Approach

Santiago Arango-Santander [1,*], Lina Serna [1], Juliana Sanchez-Garzon [1,2] and John Franco [1,3]

[1] GIOM Group, Faculty of Dentistry, Universidad Cooperativa de Colombia, Envigado 055422, Colombia; lina.sernaga@campusucc.edu.co (L.S.); juliana.sanchezga@campusucc.edu.co (J.S.-G.); john.francoa@campusucc.edu.co (J.F.)
[2] Faculty of Dentistry, CES University, Medellín 050021, Colombia
[3] Salud y Sostenibilidad Group, School of Microbiology, Universidad de Antioquia, Medellín 050010, Colombia
* Correspondence: santiago.arango@campusucc.edu.co; Tel.: +57-4-4446065

Abstract: Bacterial adhesion to surfaces is the first step in biofilm formation, which leads to the development of conditions that may compromise the health status of patients. Surface modification has been proposed to reduce bacterial adhesion to biomaterials. The objective of this work was to assess and compare *Streptococcus mutans* adhesion to the surface of biomimetically-modified stainless steel using different topographies. Stainless steel plates were modified using a soft lithography technique following a biomimetic approach. The leaves from *Colocasia esculenta*, *Crocosmia aurea* and *Salvinia molesta* were used as surface models. Silica sol was synthesized using the sol-gel method. Following a soft lithography technique, the surface of the leaves were transferred to the surface of the SS plates. Natural and modified surfaces were characterized by means of atomic force microscopy and contact angle. *Streptococcus mutans* was used to assess bacterial adhesion. Contact angle measurements showed that natural leaves are highly hydrophobic, but such hydrophobicity could not be transferred to the metallic plates. Roughness varied among the leaves and increased after transference for *C. esculenta* and decreased for *C. aurea*. In general, two of the surface models used in this investigation showed positive results for reduction of bacterial adhesion (*C. aurea* and *C. esculenta*), while the other showed an increase in bacterial adhesion (*S. molesta*). Therefore, since a biomimetic approach using natural surfaces showed opposite results, careful selection of the surface model needs to be taken into consideration.

Keywords: surface topography; bacterial adhesion; biomimetics; soft lithography; surface modification

1. Introduction

Stainless steel (SS) is a biomaterial that is highly used to manufacture devices that will be in close contact with human tissues for extended periods of time [1–3]. In the field of dentistry, particularly in orthodontics, SS is immensely used to fabricate appliances and devices, such as archwires and brackets, due to its outstanding anticorrosive properties [4–6]. However, since such devices are located within the oral cavity, they are highly susceptible to bacterial adhesion and biofilm formation due to the surface properties of this biomaterial [7–10].

Surface roughness and hydrophobicity are two of the most relevant properties involved in the process of bacterial adhesion and biofilm formation. Surface roughness promotes bacterial adhesion [11] and surface hydrophobicity allows bacterial species to adhere, colonize and grow on a surface [11,12]. Bacterial adhesion to such devices is favored by the fact that SS may have a rough surface; this adhesion will eventually lead to the formation of a mature biofilm that has the potential to cause harmful conditions to surrounding natural tissues, such as dental caries or gingivitis [13,14].

Different approaches, especially oral hygiene-related procedures, have been investigated over the years to reduce bacterial adhesion to natural and artificial surfaces [15–17]. Nonetheless, these methods have proven insufficient. An additional approach, known as surface modification, has been reported in the scientific literature in recent years. Surface modification is a vast field that includes many different chemical [18,19] and physical techniques. Topographic modifications at micro and nanometric scales is one of such physical approaches [20].

Physical surface modification techniques are divided into two large areas: top-down techniques, in which nano or microstructures are created from larger structures, and bottom-up techniques, in which larger structures are created from smaller elements [21,22]. Soft lithography belongs to the former and is a set of techniques based on self-assembly and replica molding to create micro and nano structures on the surface of materials [22,23]. Soft lithography is based upon copying and transferring the topography of a master model, which has been traditionally created using photolithography [23], to another surface. However, nature has shown, over thousands of years, that an enormous number of master models are readily available to be used for human strategies. Such inspiration in natural models is known as biomimetics [24,25]. Modified surfaces inspired by animal sources have been previously investigated [24,26], but botanical products have been scarcely used as models to modify the surface of biomaterials. Natural vegetal products, such as the leaves from Taro (*Colocasia esculenta*), Montbretia (*Crocosmia aurea*) and Giant salvinia (*Salvinia molesta*) display particular surface features, including water repellency and self-cleaning abilities, that may be interesting when considering using natural surfaces as models for surface modification [23].

Surface modification to reduce bacterial adhesion has been studied and reported in the scientific literature over the last years. Different authors have demonstrated that bacterial adhesion is reduced to physically modified surfaces [27,28]. Biomimetics has served as inspiration to other authors to emulate natural patterns, like the shark skin, and transfer them to the surface of biomaterials [29], while other investigations have shown that the topography of natural leaves reduces bacterial adhesion on SS and titanium alloy orthodontic wires [30]. However, even though the reported results are highly promising, information on using botanical sources as models to modify the surface of biomaterials is scarce and only a few plants or leaves have been reported.

Therefore, the objective of this work was to modify the surface of SS plates using the topography from three natural leaves and compare the adhesion of *Streptococcus mutans* to such modified surfaces.

2. Materials and Methods

2.1. Substrates

Stainless steel 316L (SS316L) plates (Onlinemetals.com, Seattle, WA, USA) with dimensions of 1.0 cm × 1.0 cm × 1.0 mm were used. Plates were sequentially polished using silicon carbide abrasive papers (400–1200 grit, Abracol, Colombia) and a mirror-like surface was obtained using diamond paste (0.5 µm, Leco Corporation, St. Joseph, MI, USA). SS plates were then sequentially cleaned in an ultrasonic bath using 99.8% acetone (Merck Millipore, Burlington, MA, USA), distilled water (Protokimica, Medellin, Colombia) and 99% ethanol (Merck Millipore, Burlington, MA, USA). Plates were allowed to dry in air and were divided into four groups, one of them regarded as the control group (polished SS 316L).

2.2. Master Model

The lamina of the leaves from Taro (*Colocasia esculenta*), Montbretia (*Crocosmia aurea*) and Giant salvinia (*Salvinia molesta*) were used to fabricate the master models. Such leaves were selected because they show high hydrophobicity and self-cleaning properties at simple observation without technical equipment.

2.3. Sol-Gel Synthesis

Silica sol was synthesized following the one-stage sol-gel method [31]. Tetraethylorthosilicate (TEOS) and methyltrietoxysilane (MTES) (ABCR GmbH & Co., Karlsruhe, Germany) were used as silica precursors, 0.1 N nitric acid (Merck Millipore, Burlington, MA, USA) and acetic acid (glacial, 100% v/v, Merck Millipore, Burlington, MA, USA) were used as catalyzers and absolute ethanol (99.9% v/v, Merck Millipore, Burlington, MA, USA) was used as solvent. Final silica concentration was 18 g·L^{-1}. The sol was synthesized in a thermostatic bath at 40 °C under constant stirring at 300 rpm for 3 h. It was stored at 4 °C for 24 h before using.

2.4. Soft Lithography

For the three experimental groups, the corresponding natural leaves were cut in 5.0 cm-diameter segments. These fragments were located at the bottom of silicone containers with the lamina of the leaf facing upward. Polydimethylsiloxane (PDMS, Silastic T-2, Dow Corning Corporation, Midland, MI, USA) was used to duplicate the topography of each leaf. To obtain the stamp, PDMS was prepared according to the manufacturer and was poured to cover each fragment. Polymerization for 24 h was allowed, followed by further heat treatment at 80 °C for 3 h to finish the process. PDMS stamps containing the topography from each leaf were obtained. To transfer the topography from each stamp to the corresponding SS 316L plate, a drop of 7 µL of silica sol was placed on the SS surface, the stamp was placed on top of the drop and gentle pressure was applied to distribute the sol throughout the surface. Gelation was allowed for 4 h at RT and then the stamp was removed. The plates from the experimental groups were subjected to heat treatment at 450 °C for 30 min. After this procedure, three experimental groups were obtained (one group per topography).

2.5. Surface Characterization

The natural leaves, polished SS 316L plates and transferred plates from the three experimental groups were characterized by means of atomic force microscopy (AFM, Nanosurf Easyscan 2, Nanosurf AG, Liestal, Switzerland), to determine the surface roughness, and contact angle (CA) method to assess surface hydrophobicity. For AFM acquisition, a NCLR tip (Nanosensors™, Neuchâtel, Switzerland) in tapping mode at a constant force of 48 N/m was used. AFM images were processed using AxioVision software (V 4.9.1.0, Carl Zeiss Microscopy GmbH, Jena, Germany), Image J software (1.51 J, Laboratory for Optical and Computational Instrumentation, University of Winsconsin, Madison, WI, USA) [32] and WSxM software (5.0, Nanotec Electronic and New Microscopy Laboratory, Madrid, Spain) [33]. 10 AFM images of 50 × 50 µm^2 per group were used to obtain the arithmetic average of the roughness profile (Ra) using the Gwyddion software (2.34, Department of Nanometrology, Czech Metrology Institute, Brno, Czech Republic). For surface hydrophobicity, the sessile drop method was used on 10 plates from each group. A camera (Canon EOS Rebel XS, Tokyo, Japan) and a macro lens (105 mm F2.8 EX DG OS, Sigma, Ronkonkoma, NY, USA) were used to obtain the images and the angle values were obtained using software AxioVision (V. 4.9.1.0).

2.6. Bacterial Adhesion Test

Streptococcus mutans (ATCC 25175, Microbiologics, St. Cloud, MN, USA) was used to assess bacterial adhesion to control and experimental surfaces following a previously validated protocol [30,34]. *S. mutans* was grown in Brain Heart Infusion (BHI) agar (Scharlab S.L., Barcelona, Spain) supplemented with 0.2 U/mL bacitracin (Sigma Fluka, St. Louis, MO, USA) followed by incubation for 24 h at 37 ± 1 °C. Then, *S. mutans* was cultured in peptone water for 24 h at 37 ± 1 °C. The bacterial suspension was centrifuged at 5000× g for 15 min, supernatant was discarded and the bacterial pellet was re-suspended in peptone water at 10^7 CFU/mL by measuring the nephelometric turbidity unit (NTU) (based on a calibration curve of NTU vs. CFU/mL). 15 plates from control and each experimental group were used for bacterial adhesion tests. Each plate from each group was placed at the bottom of the well of a 24-well non-treated polystyrene plate (Costar, Corning Inc., NY, USA) and 500 µL of the bacterial solution was added to cover each SS 316L plate. Polystyrene plates were incubated for 8 h at 37 ± 1 °C to allow bacterial adhesion. After this time, experimental and control plates were carefully rinsed three times with 0.9% saline solution (Corpaul, Medellin, Colombia) to remove non-adherent bacterial cells. Then, each sample was subjected to sonication (Qsonica 125, Newtown, CT, USA) at 50% power for 3 sec to quantify viable adherent bacteria. Sonicated solutions were serially diluted and 10 µL were cultured in BHI agar, by triplicate, following the drop plate method [35]. Culture plates were incubated for 48 h at 37 ± 1 °C and then Colony Forming Units (CFU) were counted.

2.7. Statistical Analyses

Comparative analysis of roughness for the natural leaves was performed by the Student's t-test for independent variables (results from *S. molesta* were excluded). Hydrophobicity results were compared using the Kruskal-Wallis H test and post-hoc analysis with the Mann Whitney U test and Bonferroni correction. Comparison of hydrophobicity and bacterial adhesion among transferred plates was performed by the one-factor Anova test and multiple comparisons through the Tukey's HSD test. Roughness results among transferred plates were compared using the Kruskal-Wallis H test and post-hoc analysis with the Mann Whitney U test and Bonferroni correction. Bivariate analysis tests were performed after previous verification of compliance with the assumptions of normality and homoscedasticity of the variances through the statistics of Shapiro Wilk and Levene, respectively. Values of $p < 0.05$ were considered statistically significant. Software SPSS (V. 25) was used for statistical analyses.

3. Results

3.1. Surface Characterization of Natural Leaves

Figure 1 shows AFM images of the polished SS 316L control plate and *C. esculenta* and *C. aurea* natural leaves. AFM images of *S. molesta* could not be obtained due to the topographical features on the surface of the leaf, which prevented the tip from making close contact with the surface.

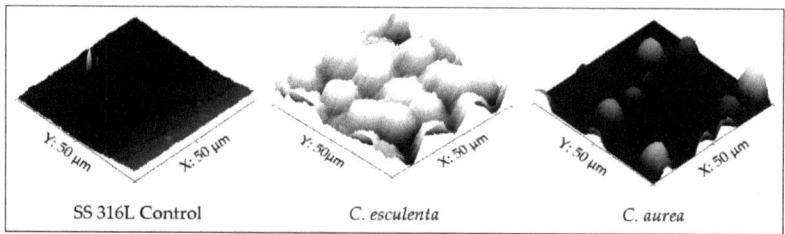

Figure 1. AFM images of a polished SS 316L (control) plate, *C. esculenta* and *C. aurea* leaves.

Contact angle measurements from the three natural leaves exhibited high hydrophobicity (contact angle > 120°). The most hydrophobic leaf was *S. molesta*, followed by *C. aurea* and *C. esculenta* (Figure 2). The differences were statistically significant ($p < 0.001$).

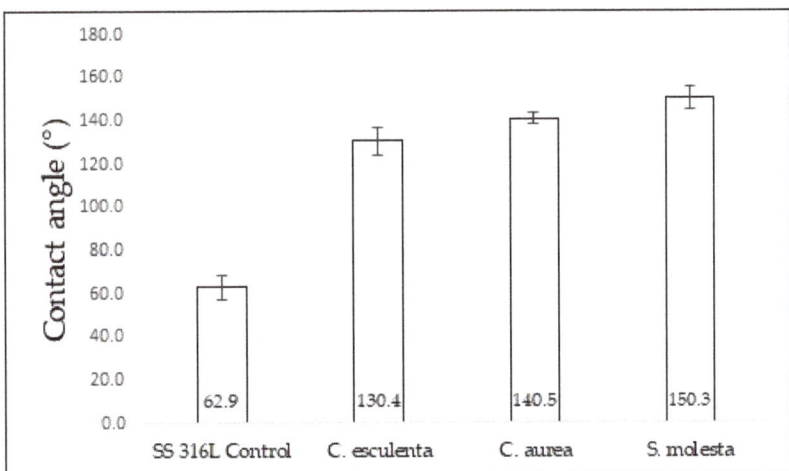

Figure 2. Contact angle measurements of control (SS 316L) surface and natural leaves.

As for roughness of the natural leaves, *C. aurea* showed higher roughness than *C. esculenta* and the difference was statistically significant ($p < 0.001$, Figure 3). As already mentioned, roughness of *S. molesta* could not be determined by AFM.

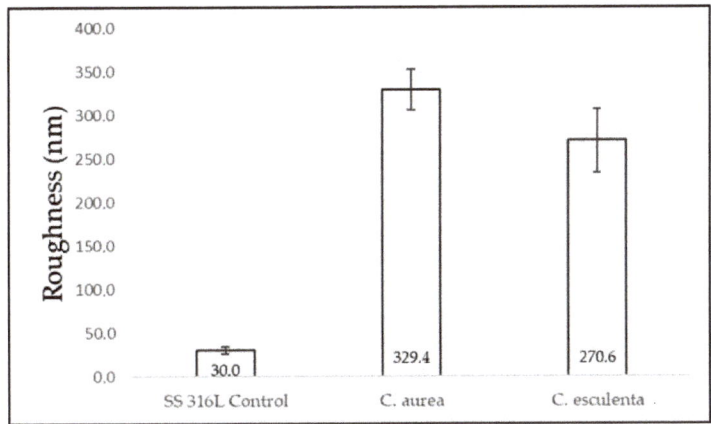

Figure 3. Average roughness of control (SS 316L) surface and natural leaves.

3.2. Surface Characterization of Modified and Control Surfaces

Regarding surface hydrophobicity of the transferred surfaces, CA measurements from plates modified with the different topographies showed higher values than the control surface. The highest CA was found for the experimental surface modified using the *C. esculenta* leaf model, followed by *S. molesta* y *C. aurea*, respectively. The difference between control and modified surfaces was statistically significant ($p < 0.001$). In addition, the difference in CA between the experimental surface modified with the *C. esculenta* leaf (highest CA value) and *C. aurea* (lowest CA value) was statistically significant ($p = 0.004$, Figure 4).

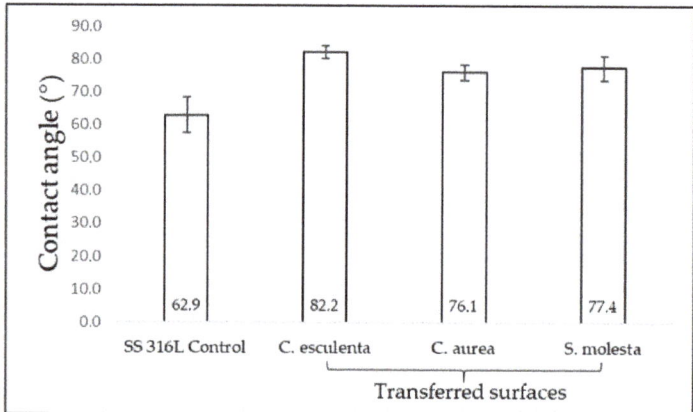

Figure 4. Contact angle measurements from control (SS 316L) and transferred (experimental) surfaces.

When comparing surface roughness from modified surfaces versus SS 316L control, the former showed higher R_a values, and the plates modified using the *C. aurea* leaf showed the highest values, followed by *C. esculenta* and SS 316L control. The difference between modified surfaces and SS 316L control was statistically significant ($v < 0.001$, Figure 5). In addition, the Ra values from the plates modified using the *C. aurea* leaf were lower than the respective natural leaf. In contrast, the Ra values from the plates modified using the *C. esculenta* leaf were higher than the respective natural leaf (data not shown). Such comparison could not be made for *S. molesta* since Ra values could not be obtained for the natural leaf as explained above.

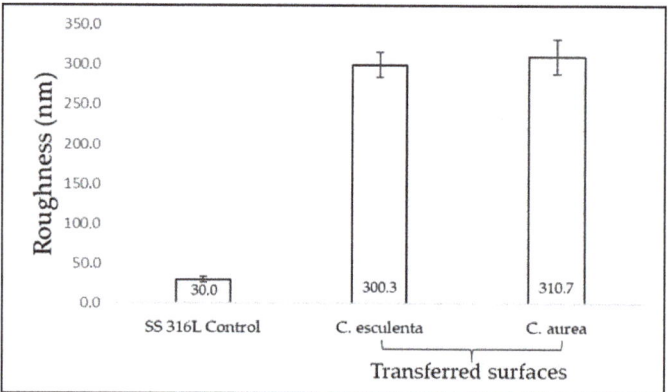

Figure 5. Average roughness of control (SS316L) and transferred (experimental) surfaces.

3.3. Evaluation of *S. mutans* Adhesion

The values from the plates modified using the *C. aurea* leaf showed the lowest adhesion ($1.3 \times 10^6 \pm 2.5 \times 10^5$ CFU/surface) when compared to control surface ($1.9 \times 10^6 \pm 2.5 \times 10^5$ CFU/surface) and the other two experimental surfaces ($1.9 \times 10^6 \pm 2.4 \times 10^5$ CFU/surface and $2.3 \times 10^6 \pm 5.0 \times 10^5$ CFU/surface for *C. esculenta* and *S. molesta*, respectively). The difference was statistically significant ($p < 0.001$). The modified surface using the *C. esculenta* leaf showed lower adhesion than the plate modified with the *S. molesta* topography. However, the values from *C. esculenta* modification and SS 316L were similar and the difference was not statistically significant (Figure 6). In addition, when comparing the *S. mutans* adhesion to the plates modified using the *S. molesta* topography versus the other treatments, including the control surface, higher values were found

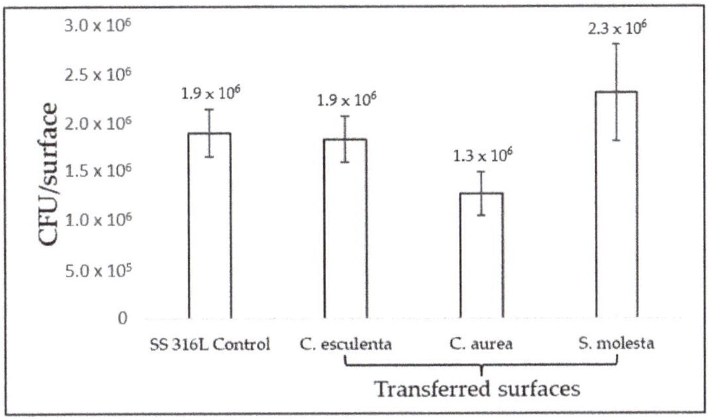

Figure 6. *S. mutans* adhesion to control (SS 316L) and transferred (experimental) surfaces.

4. Discussion

In recent years, different papers have addressed the subject of how topographic modifications on the surface of biomaterials may assist in reducing bacterial adhesion and biofilm formation [27–29]. The current investigation assessed *S. mutans* adhesion to the surface of surgical-grade stainless steel plates that were modified using different topographies following biomimetic inspiration. Natural patterns were selected based on their ability to self-clean and the apparent high hydrophobicity exhibited in their natural environment (water-repellency).

The topography of the natural leaves used as models was assessed and relevant properties were measured. They showed high hydrophobicity (130.4° for *C. esculenta*, 140.5° for *C. aurea* and 150.3° for *S. molesta*, on average). According to hydrophobicity values presented by Kim and Choi [36] and Falde et al. [37], only the *S. molesta* leaf could be classified as superhydrophobic (CA > 150°), while *C. esculenta* and *C. aurea* were classified as hydrophobic (CA between 90° and 150°). Jaggessar et al. [38] reported a contact angle between 90° and 150° for *C. esculenta*, which is in agreement with the values obtained in the present work. For comparison purposes, no values could be found for *C. aurea* and *S. molesta* in the scientific literature.

Then, a comparison between the hydrophobicity values from the natural surfaces and the values from the transferred surfaces was performed and a reduction in the contact angle measurement after the transference was found in all cases. Even though there was a reduction in hydrophobicity values, they were still higher than SS 316L. This finding may have different explanations. Biological surfaces, including natural leaves, may have protective coatings made of natural waxes that increase the hydrophobicity and such coatings could not be transferred to stainless steel plates using soft lithography [36–41]. In addition, silica sol-gel was used to transfer the topography from each leaf to polished SS 316L. Several authors [42–44] have found that when silica sol synthesized with similar TEOS:MTES ratios as the ones in the current investigation is used to coat SS surfaces, an increase in hydrophobicity is found due to the presence of methyl groups from the silica that reduce the ability of the surface to absorb water [44]. Therefore, the presence of silica may explain why the hydrophobicity values from the transferred surfaces are higher than the value from polished SS 316L. However, this effect of silica on stainless steel is not as strong as the effect that a protective wax coating has in the natural plants and leaves, hence, the values from natural sources are significantly higher than those from the transferred surfaces, which are, in turn, higher than silica-free SS 316L.

Regarding roughness, the values from the *S. molesta* leaf could not be obtained using AFM due to the topography of this natural surface consisting of multiple macrometric hair-like structures that prevented the tip from making close contact with the surface, which is necessary to obtain a correct reading. The topography of a given sample is one of the limitations exhibited by AFM, especially when the sample has steeply inclined surfaces [45], such as the topographic features shown by *S. molesta*, even at higher scales. The roughness of the remaining natural leaves (*C. aurea* and *C. esculenta*) was similar, but when comparing the roughness from the natural leaves and the transferred surfaces, an increase in roughness was observed for *C. esculenta* and a reduction was found for *C. aurea*. Such reduction in roughness may be explained by the fact that biological surfaces could have a hierarchical structure and intricate architecture [40,46] and the transfer process employed in this protocol used smooth silica sol, which may have filled some of the irregularities on the surface, hence the reduction that was observed. An explanation for the increase in roughness in the transfer of *C. esculenta* remains to be elucidated.

As for bacterial adhesion, surface roughness and hydrophobicity play a major role in how bacterial species adhere to a surface and form a biofilm. De la Pinta et al. [47] found that more abundant biofilm was formed on rougher surfaces, but such results could not be correlated when hydrophobicity was considered. Raspor et al. [48] assessed bacterial adhesion to five SS 304 surfaces to determine the influence of roughness on adhesion. They found that adhesion increases as roughness increases. Bohinc et al. [49] also obtained similar results on glass. Díaz et al. [50,51] demonstrated that roughness at the nano scale reduces bacterial adhesion, while roughness at the micro scale increases it. Xu et al. [52] confirmed such findings and explained that such reduction at the nano scale is due to the narrow space available for the bacterium and the obstacle that this represents for bacterial aggregation, which had been previously established by Hochbaum and Aizenberg [27]. These findings are conflicting with the results of the current work, since the rougher topography (*C. aurea*) showed the lower bacterial adhesion. This may be explained by the fact that, even though both the modified surface using the *C. aurea* model and the actual leaf showed higher roughness values, its apparently more organized topography and/or the size of its surface features related to the size of the bacterial species used [27] were responsible for the reduction in bacterial adhesion.

When analyzing the relation between hydrophobicity and bacterial adhesion, the higher the CA value, the lower the *S. mutans* adhesion. The most hydrophobic surface (*S. molesta*) showed an increase in bacterial adhesion, while the less hydrophobic surfaces (*C. aurea* and *C. esculenta*) exhibited lower adhesion of this bacterial species. Since it was not possible to obtain the roughness value from *S. molesta*, it is not possible to determine that the increase in bacterial adhesion is solely ascribable to its hydrophobicity, but a combination of high hydrophobicity and an apparent high roughness. It is important to notice that the difference in the relation between hydrophobicity and bacterial adhesion between the current investigation and the work by De la Pinta et al. [47] may be due to the bacterial species under evaluation, since more hydrophobic species prefer more hydrophobic surfaces. In the current work, *S. mutans* showed lower adhesion to more hydrophobic surfaces, which is in agreement with the results by Satou et al. [53], who demonstrated that *S. mutans* is a hydrophilic bacterial species that show more affinity to hydrophilic surfaces.

Adhesion to topographically modified surfaces has been addressed in the literature for a few years. Vladillo-Rodriguez et al. [54] created engineered nano surfaces and assessed bacterial adhesion. They concluded that different surface patterns caused reduction of bacterial adhesion ranging from 40% to over 95%. Bhardwaj and Webster [55] modified titanium substrates and found a 95% reduction in *Staphylococcus aureus* adhesion, a 90% reduction in *Pseudomonas aeruginosa* adhesion and a 81% reduction in *Escherichia coli* adhesion.

When modifications were based on natural models (biomimetics), Carman et al. [56] used a surface based on the sharkskin, known as Sharklet, and found a reduction in the aggregation of spores from green algae. May et al. [28], Chung et al. [29] and Reddy et al. [57]

found a reduction in bacterial adhesion to modified surfaces, using patterns from the Sharklet model, on different materials. Bixler et al. [24] evaluated anti-fouling properties of microstructures based on butterfly wings and rice leaves and obtained promising results. However, most works on surface modification using bio-inspired or biomimetic approaches are based on surfaces obtained from animal models, while plants offer many possibilities that need to be evaluated. Previous works using surface modification based on a natural leaf (*C. esculenta*) have also demonstrated a reduction in bacterial adhesion to SS and titanium surfaces [30,34]. Since *C. aurea* showed better results than *C. esculenta* for reduction in bacterial adhesion in the current work, future investigations using botanical materials as models to modify biomaterials surfaces must be continued.

5. Conclusions

Within the limitations of the current investigation, a topographic modification of the smooth surface of a metallic biomaterial showed reduction in bacterial adhesion. Three different topographies from natural leaves (*C. aurea*, *C. esculenta* and *S. molesta*) were used, but only surfaces based on *C. aurea* and *C. esculenta* models showed such effect, even though there was an increase in roughness after every transference. There were also a reduction in the hydrophobicity after the transference due to hierarchical features and protective coatings that soft lithography is incapable of transferring. The most hydrophobic surfaces showed higher bacterial adhesion, which is also related to the bacterial species used in the current investigation. The results in bacterial adhesion suggests a relation between roughness, hydrophobicity and topographic features that is relevant to reduce the adhesion of this bacterial species to the surface of SS. Such reduction is important in short term investigations because it opens new possibilities in the field of using materials and surfaces that nature has to offer to improve biomaterials for medical and dental applications. However, due to conflicting results obtained in the present work, careful attention must be given to the selection of the natural surface.

Author Contributions: Conceptualization, S.A.-S.; Data curation, J.S.-G. and J.F.; Formal analysis, J.S.-G. and J.F.; Investigation, S.A.-S. and L.S.; Methodology, S.A.-S. and L.S.; Project administration, S.A.-S.; Supervision, S.A.-S. and J.S.-G.; Writing—original draft, S.A.-S. and L.S.; Writing—review & editing, S.A.-S., J.S.-G. and J.F. All authors have read and agreed to the published version of the manuscript.

Funding: This research received no external funding.

Institutional Review Board Statement: Not applicable.

Informed Consent Statement: Not applicable.

Data Availability Statement: The data presented in this study are available on request from the corresponding author.

Acknowledgments: The authors would like to thank Claudia García from Universidad Nacional de Colombia for her assistance with the sol-gel method and Johanna Gutiérrez from Tecnoacademia for her assistance with the AFM.

Conflicts of Interest: The authors declare no conflict of interest.

References

1. Robert, M.; Ezzell, J. *Regulatory Affairs for Biomaterials and Medical Devices*, 1st ed.; McGraw Hill: New York, NY, USA, 2014.
2. Patel, N.R.; Gohil, P.P. A review on biomaterials: Scope, applications & human anatomy significance. *IJETAE* **2012**, *2*, 91–101.
3. Watts, D. Orthodontic adhesive resins. In *Orthodontic Material: Scientific and Clinical Aspects*, 1st ed.; Thieme Medical Publ Inc.: Stuttgart, Germany, 2001; pp. 202–217.
4. Oh, K.T.; Choo, S.U.; Kim, K.M.; Kim, K.N. A stainless steel bracket for orthodontic application. *Eur. J. Orthod.* **2005**, *27*, 237–244. [CrossRef]
5. Pérez, L.; Garmas, E. Mini implantes, una opción para el anclaje en ortodoncia. *Gac. Médica Espirituana* **2010**, *12*, 1–9. Available online: http://revgmespirituana.sld.cu (accessed on 10 March 2021).

6. Uribe, G.; Aristiz, J.F. Metales y Alambres De Ortodoncia. In *Ortodoncia Teoría y Clínica*, 1st ed.; Marcolud: Bogota, Colombia, 2004; pp. 226–245.
7. Ábalos, C. Adhesión bacteriana a biomateriales. *Av. Odontoestomatol.* **2005**, *21*, 347–353. [CrossRef]
8. Koch, K.; Barthlott, W. Superhydrophobic and superhydrophilic plant surfaces: An inspiration for biomimetic materials. *Philos. Trans. R. Soc. A Math. Phys. Eng. Sci.* **2009**, *367*, 1487–1509. [CrossRef]
9. Berg, J.M.; Romoser, A.; Banerjee, N.; Zebda, R.; Sayes, C.M. The relationship between pH and zeta potential of ~30 nm metal oxide nanoparticle suspensions relevant to in vitro toxicological evaluations. *Nanotoxicology* **2009**, *3*, 276–283. [CrossRef]
10. Kiremitçi-Gümü, M. Microbial adhesion to ionogenic PHEMA, PU and PP implants. *Biomaterials* **1996**, *17*, 443–449. [CrossRef]
11. Abrams, G.A.; Teixeira, A.I.; Nealey, P.F.; Murphy, C.J. Effects of substratum topography on cell behavior. *Biomim. Mater. Des.* **2002**, *33*, 91–137.
12. Zhang, X.; Wang, L.; Levänen, E. Superhydrophobic surfaces for the reduction of bacterial adhesion. *RSC Adv.* **2013**, *3*, 12003–12020. [CrossRef]
13. Pitts, N.B.; Zero, D.T.; Marsh, P.D.; Ekstrand, K.; Weintraub, J.A.; Ramos-Gomez, F.; Tagami, J.; Twetman, S.; Tsakos, G.; Ismail, A. Dental caries. *Nat. Rev. Dis. Primers* **2017**, *3*, 1–16. [CrossRef]
14. Moulis, E.; Chabadel, O.; Goldsmith, M.C.; Canal, P. Prevención de caries y ortodoncia. *EMC-Pediatría* **2008**, *43*, 1–9. [CrossRef]
15. Marsh, P.D. Are dental diseases examples of ecological catastrophes? *Microbiology* **2003**, *149*, 279–294. [CrossRef]
16. Teles, R.P.; Teles, F.R.F. Antimicrobial agents used in the control of periodontal biofilms: Effective adjuncts to mechanical plaque control? *Braz. Oral Res.* **2009**, *23*, 39–48. [CrossRef] [PubMed]
17. Bradshaw, D.J. To the control of oral biofilms. *Adv. Dent. Res.* **1997**, *11*, 176–185.
18. Hall-Stoodley, L.; Nistico, L.; Sambanthamoorthy, K.; Dice, B.; Nguyen, D.; Mershon, W.J.; Johnson, C.; Hu, F.Z.; Stoodley, P.; Ehrlich, G.D.; et al. Characterization of biofilm matrix, degradation by DNase treatment and evidence of capsule downregulation in Streptococcus pneumoniae clinical isolates. *BMC Microbiol.* **2008**, *8*, 1–16. [CrossRef] [PubMed]
19. Darouiche, R.O.; Mansouri, M.D.; Gawande, P.V.; Madhyastha, S. Antimicrobial and antibiofilm efficacy of triclosan and DispersinB® combination. *J. Antimicrob. Chemother.* **2009**, *64*, 88–93. [CrossRef]
20. Biswas, A.; Bayer, I.S.; Biris, A.S.; Wang, T.; Dervishi, E.; Faupel, F. Advances in top-down and bottom-up surface nanofabrication: Techniques, applications & future prospects. *Adv. Colloid Interface Sci.* **2012**, *170*, 2–27.
21. Arango, S.; Peláez-Vargas, A.; García, C. Coating and surface treatments on orthodontic metallic materials. *Coatings* **2012**, *3*, 1–15. [CrossRef]
22. Xia, Y.; Whitesides, G. Soft lithography. *Annu. Rev. Mater. Sci.* **1998**, *28*, 153–184. [CrossRef]
23. Whitesides, G.M.; Ostuni, E.; Jiang, X.; Ingber, D.E. Soft lithography in biology. *Annu. Rev. Biomed. Eng.* **2001**, *3*, 335–373. [CrossRef]
24. Bixler, G.D.; Theiss, A.; Bhushan, B.; Lee, S.C. Anti-fouling properties of microstructured surfaces bio-inspired by rice leaves and butterfly wings. *J. Colloid Interface Sci.* **2014**, *419*, 114–133. [CrossRef]
25. Rocha-Rangel, E. Biomimética: De la naturaleza a la creación humana. *Ciencias* **2010**, *4*, 1–8.
26. Bhadra, C.M.; Khanh Truong, V.; Pham, V.T.H.; Al Kobaisi, M.; Seniutinas, G.; Wang, J.Y.; Juodkazis, S.; Crawford, R.J.; Ivanova, E.P. Antibacterial titanium nano-patterned arrays inspired by dragonfly wings. *Sci. Rep.* **2015**, *5*, 16817. [CrossRef]
27. Hochbaum, A.; Aizenberg, J. bacteria pattern spontaneously on periodic nanostructure arrays. *Nano Lett.* **2010**, *10*, 3717–3721. [CrossRef]
28. May, R.M.; Hoffman, M.G.; Sogo, M.J.; Parker, A.E.; O'Toole, G.A.; Brennan, A.B.; Reddy, S.T. Micro-patterned surfaces reduce bacterial colonization and biofilm formation in vitro: Potential for enhancing endotracheal tube designs. *Clin. Transl. Med.* **2014**, *3*, 1–8. [CrossRef]
29. Chung, K.K.; Schumacher, J.F.; Sampson, E.M.; Burne, R.A.; Antonelli, P.J.; Brennan, A.B. Impact of engineered surface microtopography on biofilm formation of Staphylococcus aureus. *Biointerphases* **2007**, *2*, 89–94. [CrossRef]
30. Arango-Santander, S.; Gonzalez, C.; Aguilar, A.; Cano, A.; Castro, S.; Sanchez-Garzon, J.; Franco, J. Assessment of streptococcus mutans adhesion to the surface of biomimetically-modified orthodontic archwires. *Coatings* **2020**, *10*, 201. [CrossRef]
31. Arango-Santander, S.; Freitas, S.; Pelaez-Vargas, A.; Garcia, C. Silica sol-gel patterned surfaces based on dip-pen nanolithography and microstamping: A comparison in resolution and throughput. *Key Eng. Mater.* **2016**, *720*, 264–268. [CrossRef]
32. Schneider, C.A.; Rasband, W.S.; Eliceiri, K.W. NIH image to ImageJ: 25 years of image analysis. *Nat. Methods* **2012**, *9*, 671–675. [CrossRef] [PubMed]
33. Horcas, I.; Fernández, R.; Gómez-Rodríguez, J.M.; Colchero, J.; Gómez-Herrero, J.; Baro, A.M. WSXM: A software for scanning probe microscopy and a tool for nanotechnology. *Rev. Sci. Instrum.* **2007**, *78*, 1–8. [CrossRef] [PubMed]
34. Arango-Santander, S.; Pelaez-Vargas, A.; Freitas, S.; García, C. Surface modification by combination of dip-pen nanolithography and soft lithography for reduction of bacterial adhesion. *J. Nanotech.* **2018**, *2018*, 1–10. [CrossRef]
35. Naghili, H.; Tajik, H.; Mardani, K.; Razavi Rouhani, S.M.; Ehsani, A.; Zare, P. Validation of drop plate technique for bacterial enumeration by parametric and nonparametric tests. *Vet. Res. Forum* **2013**, *4*, 179–183.
36. Kim, J.; Choi, S.O. Superhydrophobicity. Waterproof and water repellent textiles and clothing. In *The Textile Institute Book Series*; Woodhead Publishing: Sawston, UK, 2018; pp. 267–297.
37. Falde, E.; Yohe, S.; Colson, Y.; Grinstaff, M. Superhydrophobic materials for biomedical applications. *Biomaterials* **2016**, *104*, 87–103. [CrossRef]

38. Jaggessar, A.; Shahali, H.; Mathew, A.; Yarlagadda, P. Bio-mimicking nano and micro-structured surface fabrication for antibacterial properties in medical implants. *J. Nanobiotech.* **2017**, *15*, 1–20. [CrossRef]
39. Burton, Z.; Bhushan, B. Surface characterization and adhesion and friction properties of hydrophobic leaf surfaces. *Ultramicroscopy* **2006**, *106*, 709–719. [CrossRef] [PubMed]
40. Grewal, H.; Cho, I.; Yoon, E. The role of bio-inspired hierarchical structures in wetting. *Bioinspiration Biomim.* **2015**, *10*, 026009. [CrossRef] [PubMed]
41. Bhushan, B. Biomimetics: Lessons from nature-An overview. *Philos. Trans. R. Soc. A* **2009**, *367*, 1445–1486. [CrossRef] [PubMed]
42. Santos, O.; Nylander, T.; Rosmaninho, R.; Rizzo, G.; Yiantsios, S.; Andritsos, N.; Karabelas, A.; Müller-Steinhagen, H.; Melo, L.; Boulangé-Petermann, L.; et al. Modified stainless steel surfaces targeted to reduce fouling—Surface characterization. *J. Food Eng.* **2004**, *64*, 63–79. [CrossRef]
43. Hosseinalipour, S.M.; Ershad-langroudi, A.; Hayati, A.N.; Nabizade-Haghighi, A.M. Characterization of sol-gel coated 316L stainless steel for biomedical applications. *Prog. Org. Coat.* **2010**, *67*, 371–374. [CrossRef]
44. Yang, H.; Pi, P.; Cai, Z.Q.; Wen, X.; Wang, X.; Cheng, J.; Yang, Z. Facile preparation of super-hydrophobic and super-oleophilic silica film on stainless steel mesh via sol-gel process. *Appl. Surf. Sci.* **2010**, *256*, 4095–4102. [CrossRef]
45. Haßler-Grohne, W.; Hüser, D.; Klaus-Peter, J.; Frase, C.; Bosse, H. Current limitations of SEM and AFM metrology for the characterization of 3D nanostructures. *Meas. Sci. Technol.* **2011**, *22*, 1–8. [CrossRef]
46. Xiang, Y.; Huang, S.; Huang, T.; Dong, A.; Cao, D.; Li, H.; Xue, Y.; Lv, P.; Duan, H. Superrepellency of underwater hierarchical structures on salvinia leaf. *Proc. Natl. Acad. Sci. USA* **2020**, *117*, 2282–2287. [CrossRef] [PubMed]
47. De-la-Pinta, I.; Cobos, M.; Ibarretxe, J.; Montoya, E.; Eraso, E.; Guraya, T.; Quindós, G. Effect of biomaterials hydrophobicity and roughness on biofilm development. *J. Mater. Sci. Mater. Med.* **2019**, *30*, 77. [CrossRef]
48. Raspor, P.; Bohinc, K.; Dražić, G.; Fink, R.; Oder, M.; Jevšnik, M.; Nipič, D. Available surface dictates microbial adhesion capacity. *Inter. J. Adhes. Adhes.* **2014**, *50*, 265–272.
49. Bohinc, K.; Dražić, G.; Abram, A.; Jevšnik, M.; Jeršek, B.; Nipič, D.; Kurinčič, M.; Raspor, P. Metal surface characteristics dictate bacterial adhesion capacity. *Inter. J. Adhes. Adhes.* **2016**, *68*, 39–46. [CrossRef]
50. Díaz, C.; Schilardi, P.; Salvarezza, R.; Fernández Lorenzo de Mele, M. Nano/microscale order affects the early stages of biofilm formation on metal surfaces. *Langmuir* **2007**, *23*, 11206–11210. [CrossRef] [PubMed]
51. Diaz, C.; Schilardi, P.; dos Santos Claro, P.C.; Salvarezza, R.C.; Fernandez Lorenzo de Mele, M. Submicron trenches reduce the Pseudomonas fluorescens colonization rate on solid surfaces. *Appl. Mater. Interfaces* **2009**, *1*, 136–143. [CrossRef]
52. Xu, L.C.; Siedlecki, C.A. Submicron-textured biomaterial surface reduces staphylococcal bacterial adhesion and biofilm formation. *Acta Biomater.* **2012**, *8*, 72–81. [CrossRef]
53. Satou, J.; Fukunaga, A.; Satou, N.; Shintani, H.; Okuda, K. Streptococcal adherence on various restorative materials. *J. Dent. Res.* **1988**, *67*, 588–591. [CrossRef]
54. Vadillo-Rodríguez, V.; Guerra-García-Mora, A.; Perera-Costa, D.; Gónzalez-Martín, M.; Fernández-Calderón, M. Bacterial response to spatially organized microtopographic surface patterns with nanometer scale roughness. *Colloids Surf. B Biointerfaces* **2018**, *169*, 340–347. [CrossRef]
55. Bhardwaj, G.; Webster, T.J. Reduced bacterial growth and increased osteoblast proliferation on titanium with a nanophase TiO_2 surface treatment. *Inter. J. Nanomed.* **2017**, *12*, 363–369. [CrossRef] [PubMed]
56. Carman, M.; Estes, T.; Feinberg, A.; Schumacher, J.; Wilkerson, W.; Wilson, L.; Callow, M.; Callow, J.; Brennan, A. Engineered antifouling microtopographies-Correlating wettability with cell attachment. *Biofouling* **2006**, *22*, 11–21. [CrossRef] [PubMed]
57. Reddy, S.; Chung, K.; McDaniel, C.; Darouiche, R.; Landman, J.; Brennan, A. Micropatterned surfaces for reducing the risk of catheter-associated urinary tract infection: An in vitro study on the effect of sharklet micropatterned surfaces to inhibit bacterial colonization and migration of uropathogenic escherichia coli. *J. Endourol.* **2011**, *25*, 1547–1552. [CrossRef] [PubMed]

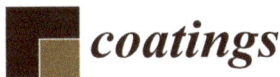

Article

Coating of a Sand-Blasted and Acid-Etched Implant Surface with a pH-Buffering Agent after Vacuum-UV Photofunctionalization

Chang-Joo Park [1,†], Jae Hyung Lim [2,†], Marco Tallarico [3], Kyung-Gyun Hwang [1], Hyook Choi [1], Gyu-Jang Cho [1], Chang Kim [1], Il-Seok Jang [4], Ju-Dong Song [4], Amy M. Kwon [5], Sang Ho Jeon [6] and Hyun-Kyung Park [7,*]

[1] Division of Oral and Maxillofacial Surgery, Department of Dentistry, College of Medicine, Hanyang University, Seoul 04763, Korea; fastchang@hanyang.ac.kr (C.-J.P.); hkg@hanyang.ac.kr (K.-G.H.); chlgur3@nate.com (H.C.); chogu@hanmail.net (G.-J.C.); himychang0@naver.com (C.K.)
[2] Division of Oral and Maxillofacial Surgery, Department of Dentistry, Korea University Ansan Hospital, Ansan 15355, Korea; surgidenta@gmail.com
[3] Department of Periodontology and Implantology, University of Sassari, 7100 Sassari, Italy; me@studiomarcotallarico.it
[4] Osstem R&D Center, Seoul 07789, Korea; microart@osstem.com (I.-S.J.); jud@osstem.com (J.-D.S.)
[5] Biostatistic Core, Medicine-Engineering-Bio (MEB) Global Development Research Centre, Hanyang University, Seoul 04763, Korea; amykwon@hanyang.ac.kr
[6] Department of Oral and Maxillofacial Surgery, Korea University Anam Hospital, Seoul 02841, Korea; junsang@korea.ac.kr
[7] Division of Neonatology, Department of Paediatrics, College of Medicine, Hanyang University, Seoul 04763, Korea
* Correspondence: neopark@hanyang.ac.kr; Tel.: +82-2-2290-8391
† These two authors contributed equally to this work.

Received: 24 September 2020; Accepted: 28 October 2020; Published: 28 October 2020

Abstract: Ultraviolet (UV) photofunctionalization can reset the biological aging of titanium after the preparation and storage of dental implants by transforming hydrophobic titanium surfaces into superhydrophilic surfaces. Blood clot formation around the implant can initialize and promote the healing process at the bone–implant interface. The aim of this study is to evaluate and compare the capabilities of surface wettability and blood clotting of implants with a conventional sand-blasted and acid-etched surface (SA), a sand-blasted and acid-etched surface with vacuum-UV treatment (SA + VUV), and a sand-blasted and acid-etched surface coated with a pH-buffering agent after vacuum-UV treatment (SA + VUV + BS). Static and dynamic tests for surface wettability and blood clotting were performed in vitro for SA + VUV and SA + VUV + BS ($n = 5$), while hemostasis resulting from blood clotting was evaluated in vivo for SA, SA +VUV, and SA + VUV + BS ($n = 4$). A Kruskal–Wallis test showed statistically significant differences ($p < 0.05$) in all tests, with the exception of in vitro test of static blood clotting. VUV treatment is therefore effective at making an SA surface superhydrophilic as an alternative to routine UV-C radiation. The addition of a pH-buffering agent to SA + VUV also improved surface wettability and blood clotting, which are crucial for successful osseointegration.

Keywords: blood clotting; dental implants; hydrophilicity; titanium; ultraviolet rays

1. Introduction

Titanium has been widely used for dental and orthopedic restoration and reconstruction due to its biocompatibility, resistance to corrosion, and mechanical properties. Titanium oxidizes easily, forming a thin (1–5 nm), stable, and passive layer that is self-limiting and protects the surface of the metal from further oxidation [1]. This titanium dioxide (TiO_2) surface layer is considered to be responsible for its effective biological performance due to the transfer of calcium and phosphorus ions from the bone matrix within the TiO_2 layer [2]. However, significant reductions in osseointegration and other biological capabilities of titanium occur over time as surface carbon increases because of an unavoidable deposition of carbon from the atmosphere on the TiO_2 layer in a form of hydrocarbon [3]. This phenomenon is defined as the biological aging of titanium, and the ability of titanium surfaces to attract proteins and osteogenic cells decreases in a time-dependent manner [4]. Another notable change in titanium surfaces with time is the disappearance of hydrophilicity. Immediately after processing, titanium surfaces exhibit a contact angle of water of 0 or less than 5 degrees, and such surfaces are called superhydrophilic [4–7]. This feature gradually attenuates and becomes hydrophobic in 2 and 4 weeks, with a contact angle of greater than 40 and 60 degrees, respectively.

Surface treatment is used to modify dental implant surface topography and energy, resulting in improved wettability, increased cell proliferation and growth, and accelerated osseointegration [1,8,9]. Surface treatment can be achieved by an additive or subtractive technique [9]. The subtractive technique either removes or roughens a layer of core material, as typified by a sand-blasted and acid-etched (SA) surface. In the addictive technique, other materials or chemical agents are added superficially to the surface of the titanium through coating, such as titanium plasma spraying, hydroxyapatite coating, calcium phosphate coating, and other biomimetic coating. Drilling prior to implant placement causes bone tissue to undergo trauma similar to a fracture. The site becomes relatively hypoxic, and the extracellular pH becomes acidic. In such conditions, bone marrow stromal cells exhibit reduced alkaline phosphatase (ALP) activity and collagen synthesis, both of which are important in bone formation and osseointegration [10]. Glycolysis and DNA synthesis of osteoblasts are also found to be affected by acidic conditions [11]. Platelet aggregation, which is a critical step in blood clot formation or thrombogenesis, is also reduced by extracellular acidosis, as mediated by the calcium ion entry pathway [12]. Formation of a sufficient blood clot offers a direct and stable link at the bone-to-implant interface and plays an important role in thrombogenic responses and osseointegration [13]. Moreover, a relationship was found between various implant surface and the extent of the fibrin clot [14].

In our previous study, a novel SA surface coated with a pH-buffering agent after vacuum-UV (VUV) treatment was introduced [15,16]. This surface was closely associated with greater affinity for proteins, cells, and platelets, which promoted rapid and stable blood clotting, thrombogenesis, and osseointegration. The purpose of the present study was to evaluate and compare the surface wettability and blood clotting abilities of various implant surfaces, including a conventional SA surface (SA), an SA surface with VUV treatment (SA + VUV), and an SA surface coated with a pH-buffering agent after VUV treatment (SA + VUV + BS), by in vitro and in vivo analyses.

2. Materials and Methods

2.1. Preparation of Implant Fixtures

Implant fixtures of commercially pure titanium (grade IV) were prepared as SA, SA + VUV (TS III SA, Osstem, Seoul, Korea), and SA + VUV + BS (TS III SOI, Osstem) for use in this study. As shown in Figure 1a,b, the surface roughness of the implant fixtures were measured to be 2.5 ± 0.5 μm of R_a value [15], and VUV treatment for photofunctionalization was achieved by exposing an implant fixture to low-pressure mercury-arc lamps emitting UV-C and VUV in UV ozone cleaner for 1 h. Coating the implant surface with a pH-buffering agent, comprising both of positively and negatively charged ionic groups, with 7.31 of pKa value at 37 °C [15,16], was supplemented for better superhydrophilicity (Figure 1c).

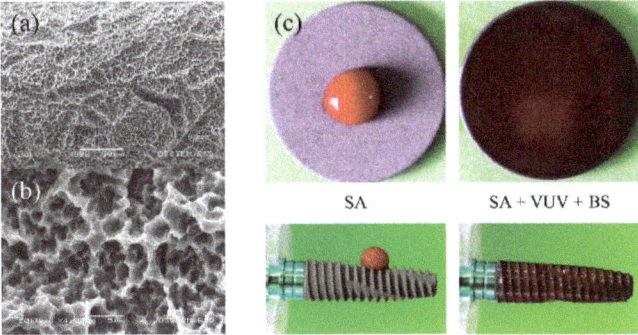

Figure 1. Morphologic observation of a sand-blasted and acid-etched (SA) surface by scanning electron microscope (SEM) at ×500 (**a**) and ×4000 magnification (**b**); (**c**) Comparison of contact angles of defibrinated sheep blood on titanium discs and implant fixtures, respectively. SA, a conventional SA surface; SA + VUV + BS, an SA surface coated with a pH-buffering agent after vacuum-UV treatment.

2.2. In Vitro Tests

2.2.1. Static Surface Wettability

Heparinized sheep blood was filled in a dish 3.5 cm in diameter to a depth of 2 to 3 cm. Implant fixtures of SA + VUV and SA + VUV + BS ($n = 5$, respectively) were immersed in blood up to the uppermost discontinuation of apical threads, and the time to reach the top of the implant fixture was recorded to calculate the wetting velocity. The time was not counted from the apex of the implant fixture, because the presence of discontinuation of apical threads caused blood absorption to stop abruptly.

2.2.2. Dynamic Surface Wettability

To simulate the clinical situations of implant fixture installation, holes were made in a transparent acrylic plate to secure visibility, according to the manufacturer's drilling protocol for hard bone density using a 122 Taper Kit (Osstem). A 130 μM sample of defibrinated sheep blood was placed into each hole of the acrylic plate, and the implant fixtures of SA + VUV and SA + VUV + BS ($n = 5$, respectively) were dipped into the hole by a push–pull gauge (MX-500N, Imada Co., Tokyo, Japan) at a speed of 50 mm/min, and the times when the blood reached up to the 2 mm and 4 mm points of the central axis of the fixture above the horizontal plate, respectively, were recorded (Figure 2).

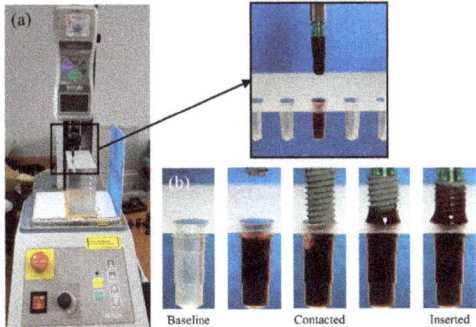

Figure 2. In vitro test of dynamic surface wettability: (**a**) a transparent acrylic plate with implant holes and the implant fixture in a push–pull gauge; (**b**) baseline, contact of the implant fixture with the blood, and whole insertion of implant fixture into the hole.

2.2.3. Static Blood Clotting

The implant fixtures of SA + VUV and SA + VUV + BS, 11.5 mm long with 4.5 mm diameter (n = 5, respectively), were dipped up to their ends in a dish 3.5 cm in diameter filled with 3 mL of non-heparinized sheep blood. The weight (g) of the blood clot around the implant fixture was measured at 5 min, 7.5 min, 10 min, and 12.5 min, respectively.

2.2.4. Dynamic Blood Clotting

This model for active blood clotting was designed to simulate continuous blood supply by capillaries. The SA + VUV and SA + VUV + BS implant fixtures, which were 10 mm long with a 4.0 mm diameter (n = 5), were inserted with 5 N cm of pre-set insertion torque into a modified Eppendorf tube, which was connected to a syringe pump infusing the sheep blood, mixed with 1 IU/mL heparin, on the bottom at 37 °C. After 30 min of blood supply at an infusion rate of 0.05 mL/min, the time (min) until blood ceased dropping by blood clot formation around the implant fixture and the volume (mL) of blood, which was collected in the underlying 15 mL tube below the Eppendorf tube, were measured.

2.3. In Vivo Test

A beagle dog mandible model was used. All procedures were conducted with the approval of the Ethics Committee of Animal Experimentation of the Institutional Animal Care and Use Committee (CRONEX-IACUC 20191002; Cronex, Hwasung, Korea) according to the guidelines of Animal Research: Reporting in Vivo Experiments (ARRIVE).

Four female beagles 18 months of age were subjected to bilateral extraction of their mandibular premolars and the first molar under general anesthesia. The anesthetic protocol for all surgical procedures included a 1 mL intramuscular injection with a 15 mg/kg dose of tiletamine/zolazepam (Zoletil 50, Virbac, Seoul, Korea) and 5 mg/kg xylazine (Rompun, Bayer Korea, Seoul, Korea). After local anesthesia, a full-thickness mucoperiosteal flap was raised adjacent to the mandibular premolars and molars (Figure 3). Teeth were hemisected under copious irrigation with a small fissure bur. Extractions were performed with elevators and forceps. Flaps were closed with single interrupted sutures. Postoperative care protocol included antibiotics and pain control. During this interval, all dogs were maintained on a soft diet and water ad libitum.

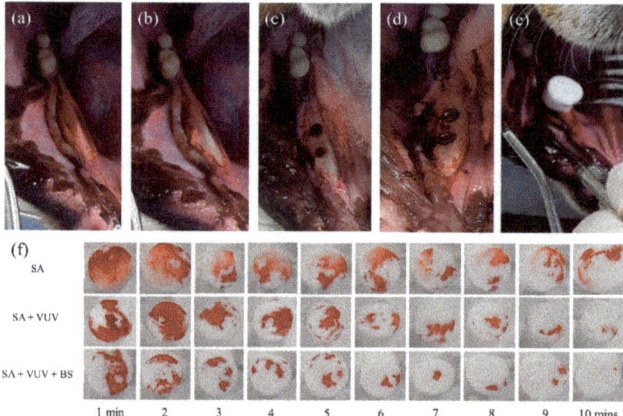

Figure 3. In vivo test of blood clotting: (**a**) incision and flap reflection; (**b**) alveolar ridge flattening; (**c**) preparation of implant holes; (**d**) implant fixture placement; (**e**) cotton pellet application for bleeding absorption; (**f**) pattern of cotton pellets according to time. SA, a conventional SA surface; SA + VUV, an SA surface with vacuum-UV treatment; SA + VUV + BS, an SA surface coated with a pH-buffering agent after vacuum-UV treatment.

Three months after the extractions, surgical placement of dental implants was performed in the healed extraction sites under sterile conditions. After local anesthesia, a full-thickness flap was elevated to expose the alveolar ridge, and the irregular alveolar crestal was flattened. Sequential drillings were performed for consecutive implant sites, which were larger than the implant fixture, using a guide drill, 2.2 mm twist drill, 3.0 mm taper drill, 4.0 mm taper drill, and 6.0 mm ultra-taper drill. A total of 12 implant fixtures of SA, SA + VUV, and SA + VUV + BS, 8.5 mm long with a 3.5 mm diameter, were placed bilaterally with 35 N cm of pre-set insertion torque. Whole bleeding from the gap between the hole and implant fixture was socked in a cotton pellet until 10 min after implant placement, and the weight (g) of the cotton pellet was measured every minute to evaluate the potential of the blood clotting of the implant fixtures. All experimental animals were sacrificed after the surgery by an intravenous overdose of potassium chloride.

2.4. Statistical Analysis

Due to a small sample size, we performed a Kruskal–Wallis test, which is a nonparametric comparison of the difference of the means without a normality assumption, to examine the differences between SA + VUV and S + VUV + BS in vitro and among SA, SA + VUV and SA + VUV + BS in vivo, with a statistical significance of $p < 0.05$ at $\alpha = 0.05$. All statistical analyses were performed using SAS, version 9.4 (SAS Inc., Cary, NC, USA).

3. Results

3.1. In Vitro Tests

3.1.1. Static Surface Wettability

The lengths of time before the blood reached the top of the implant fixture were 43.3 ± 8.3 min and 3.8 ± 0.3 min in SA + VUV and SA + VUV + BS, respectively, and a statistically significant difference ($p < 0.05$) between the two was evident (Figure 4a).

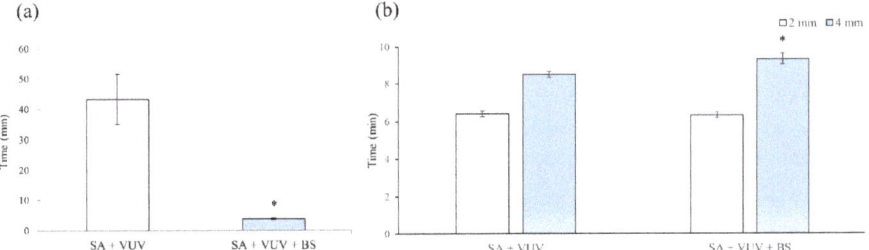

Figure 4. In vitro test of static and dynamic surface wettability: (**a**) time (min) to reach the top of the implant fixture; (**b**) time (min) to reach 2 mm and 4 mm above the horizontal plate, respectively. SA + VUV, an SA surface with vacuum-UV treatment; SA + VUV + BS, an SA surface coated with a pH-buffering agent after vacuum-UV treatment. Mean ± SD, * $p < 0.05$ by Kruskal–Wallis test.

3.1.2. Dynamic Surface Wettability

The lengths of time before the blood reached 2 mm above the horizontal plate were 6.4 ± 0.1 min and 6.3 ± 0.2 min, and for 4 mm above the horizontal plate, they were 8.5 ± 0.2 min and 9.3 ± 0.3 min in SA + VUV and SA + VUV + BS, respectively. A statistically significant difference ($p < 0.05$) between SA + VUV and SA + VUV + BS was only found for the time before the blood reached 4 mm above the horizontal plate (Figure 4b).

3.1.3. Static Blood Clotting

In SA + VUV, the weights of the blood clot formed around the implant fixture, which were measured at 5 min, 7.5 min, 10 min, and 12.5 min after immersing the implant fixture in the blood, were 0.04 ± 0.01 g, 0.09 ± 0.03 g, 0.23 ± 0.06 g, and 0.39 ± 0.16 g, respectively. In SA + VUV + BS, the weights were 0.07 ± 0.03 g, 0.12 ± 0.02 g, 0.39 ± 0.20 g, and 0.61 ± 0.18 g, respectively, and no statistically significant differences were measured between SA + VUV and SA + VUV + BS at any time ($p > 0.05$).

3.1.4. Dynamic Blood Clotting

The times for complete hemostasis were 19.0 ± 0.4 min and 8.1 ± 1.2 min in SA + VUV and SA + VUV + BS, respectively, and there was a statistically significant difference between SA + VUV and SA + VUV + BS ($p < 0.01$, Figure 5a). In addition, the volumes of the blood collected in the underlying tube were 8.27 ± 0.36 mL and 3.64 ± 0.99 mL in SA + VUV and SA + VUV + BS, respectively, with a statistically significant difference ($p < 0.01$, Figure 5b) evident between SA + VUV and SA + VUV + BS.

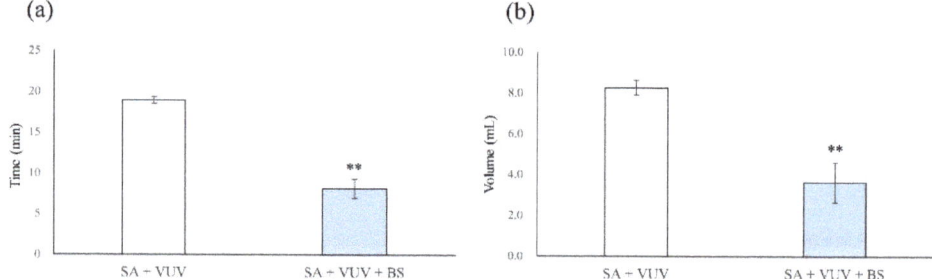

Figure 5. In vitro test of dynamic blood clotting: (**a**) time (min) until complete hemostasis; (**b**) volume (mL) of the blood collected in the underlying tube. SA + VUV, an SA surface with vacuum-UV treatment; SA + VUV + BS, an SA surface coated with a pH-buffering agent after vacuum-UV treatment. Mean ± SD, ** $p < 0.01$ by Kruskal–Wallis test.

3.2. In Vivo Test

Among SA, SA + VUV, and SA + VUV + BS, there were statistically significant differences in the weights of the whole blood absorbed in the cotton pellet measured at 5 min, 6 min, and 7 min ($p < 0.01$, Figure 6). Summary statistics of this study are shown in Table 1.

Table 1. Summary Statistics of this Study.

Tests	Categories	Groups	N	χ^2	DF	p Value
In vitro	Static surface wettability	SA + VUV vs. SA + VUV + BS	5	3.8571	1	0.0495 *
	Dynamic surface wettability	SA + VUV vs. SA + VUV + BS	5	-	-	-
	2 mm	-	-	0.4839	1	0.4867
	4 min	-	-	4.5000	1	0.0339 *
	Static blood clotting	SA + VUV vs. SA + VUV + BS	5	-	-	-
	5 min	-	-	2.3333	1	0.1266
	7.5 min	-	-	1.1905	1	0.2752
	10 min	-	-	2.3333	1	0.1266
	12.5 min	-	-	1.1905	1	0.2752
	Dynamic blood clotting	SA + VUV vs. SA + VUV + BS	5	-	-	-
	Time	-	-	12.9630	2	0.0015 **
	Volume	-	-	12.5448	2	0.0019 **
In vivo	Blood clotting	SA vs. SA + VUV vs. SA + VUV + BS	4	9.8462	2	0.0073 **

DF: degrees of freedom, N: number of samples, SA: a conventional SA surface; SA + VUV: an SA surface with vacuum-UV treatment; SA + VUV + BS: an SA surface coated with a pH-buffering agent after vacuum-UV treatment. * $p < 0.05$ and ** $p < 0.01$ by Kruskal–Wallis test.

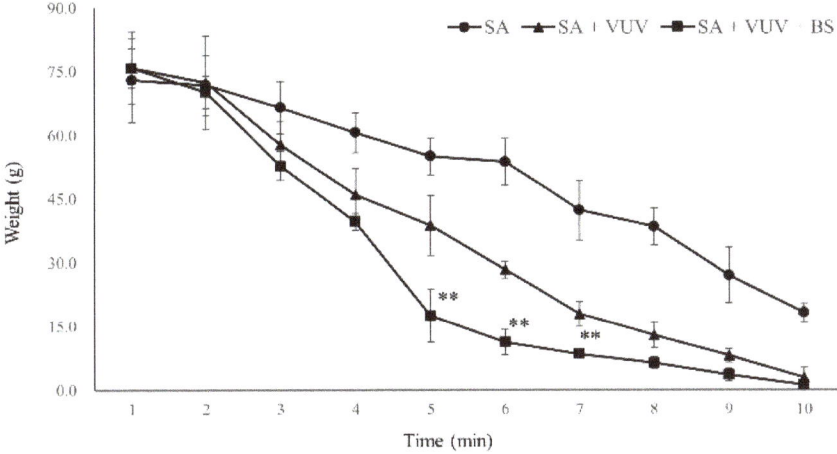

Figure 6. In vivo test of blood clotting. Weight (g) of the whole blood absorbed in the cotton pellet measured from each implant site according to time. SA, a conventional SA surface; SA + VUV, an SA surface with vacuum-UV treatment; SA + VUV + BS, an SA surface coated with a pH-buffering agent after vacuum-UV treatment. Mean ± SD, ** $p < 0.01$ by Kruskal–Wallis test.

4. Discussion

UV photofunctionalization, a method of modifying titanium surfaces after UV treatment that includes altering the physicochemical properties and enhancing biocompatibilities, has been proposed to reset the biological aging of titanium [7]. After treatment with UV radiation, the TiO_2 layer of a titanium surface incorporated with hydrocarbons became remarkably hydrophilic or superhydrophilic. The amount of surface carbon is known to vary depending on the age of the surface and reportedly can increase to approximately 60% to 70% of surface atomic components. UV treatment cleans such carbon-contaminated titanium surfaces, reducing the carbon percentage to less than 20% and concurrently increasing the level of osseointegration [7]. In the UV spectrum, both UV-A and UV-C convert biologically aged titanium surfaces from hydrophobic to superhydrophilic, but only UV-C (200–280 nm) is known to effectively reduce surface carbon to a level equivalent to a new surface and enhance bioactivity [17]. UV-C is capable of removing hydrocarbon from a TiO_2 layer of titanium by direct photodecomposition, which is more effective than photocatalysis by UV-A [18]. In our study, all implant fixtures were photofunctionalized by UV-C and VUV (100–200 nm), and the radical removal of hydrocarbon from TiO_2 layer of titanium could provide more superhydrophilicity [15,19]. VUV is rapidly absorbed by water in the atmosphere and is therefore capable of generating various reactive oxygen species by breaking hydrogen bonds in water molecules via hydrolysis [19]. VUV-initiated hydrolysis is an efficient method of obtaining hydroxide or hydroxyl groups on a TiO_2 layer that provides persistent superhydrophilicity [20,21]. Since VUV treatment tends to generate more ozone in the atmosphere and hydroxyl radicals in water [19], it should be strictly limited in only laboratory or factory, not clinical, settings.

To accelerate bone healing and improve bone anchorage to an implant, the bone/implant interface can be improved topographically and biochemically by incorporating inorganic phases, such as calcium phosphate, and organic molecules, such as proteins, enzymes or peptides, on or into a TiO_2 layer [22–25]. Nanostructured implant surfaces, which have an extensive surface area, high surface free energy, and wettability, seem capable of modifying the host tissue response [9]. SA implant surfaces have demonstrated predictable clinical results and are regarded as standard implant surface [10,26–29]. The superhydrophilicity of SA + VUV + BS, which was previously found on the flat surface of disks [15], was confirmed in our test of static surface wettability. As the ability to attract blood near to the top of the implant fixture (approximately 4 mm above the horizontal plate in our study) is what most clinicians ultimately prefer to check in a clinical setting, we added a new dynamic test of surface wettability to compare the wetting velocities of SA + VUV and SA + VUV + BS in more detail. Since SA is a dry surface that has not been in contact with any liquid, the surface wettability of SA + VUV + BS might be significantly superior to that of SA solely by the effect of the pH-buffering agent of SA + VUV + BS itself. However, given that implant fixtures are placed with dry surfaces or without any additional hydration in real clinical situations, we chose a naïve SA, rather than an SA hydrated in solution, as a control [30]. A more hydrophilic surface was previously found to be closely related to superior and faster osseointegration [30,31]. Furthermore, surface wettability is known to alter the biological responses of implant surfaces with respect to the adhesion of proteins and other molecules, as well as cell interactions [32].

As blood clot formation signals the beginning of the healing process, the interaction between an implant and blood is considered important for the successful osseointegration of titanium implants after implantation [33]. Blood clot formation on rough titanium surfaces can induce cell recruitment and stimulate wound healing [34], and it has been revealed that both preosteoblasts and osteoblasts can attach to an implant surface covered by platelets and fibrin, where they differentiate under the stimulation of osteogenic factors and cytokines released from the peri-implant blood clot [35,36]. The formation of blood clots on the implant with various implant surfaces is believed to be a crucial factor in effective fibrin retention and may critically affect bone healing and osseointegration by influencing macromolecule transport, cell behavior, and contact/distant osteogenesis [34]. In a test of static blood clotting, the SA + VUV + BS showed superior blood absorption around the implant fixtures compared with SA + VUV, but not to statistically significant degree. This indicates that an SA surface photofunctionalized with VUV has at least an equal ability in blood clotting. We designed new experiments to confirm the blood clotting by hemostasis of continuous capillary bleedings to simulate real clinical situations as accurately as possible. In a test of in vitro dynamic blood clotting, the clots formed significantly faster, and the total volume of blood collecting through the gap between holes and implant fixture to hemostasis was significantly less in SA + VUV + BS than in SA + VUV. An in vivo test also showed a significant difference in the total weight of bleeding between the overprepared hole and an implant fixture among SA, SA + VUV, and SA + VUV + BS. This suggests that SA + VUV + BS can induce faster blood clot formation around the implant surface, leading to more effective interaction of the bone-to-implant interface for osseointegration. In a clinical respect, these features of SA + VUV + BS are important in visualizing the surgical site and simultaneous guided bone regeneration, which is frequently indicated for the adequate quantity and quality of peri-implant tissues for more aesthetic and functional results [37], because rapid blood clotting is closely associated with the stabilization of grafting material and the barrier membrane. Finally, SA + VUV could be an alternative to SA + VUV + BS to SA with respect to the potential for blood clot formation on implant surfaces.

During implant drilling in the bone, which produces a weakly acidic condition, a pH buffer may help keep the pH constant [38]. As a coating material, the pH-buffering agent appears to control the release of the inflammatory mediators [9] and enhance the conditions for osteoblast activity [15] by keeping the pH constant or at least preventing significant changes. The activity of platelets in blood clotting and both the activity of osteoblasts and the level of ALP for bone making are also inhibited by extracellular acidosis [11]. SA + VUV + BS could maximize the activity of platelets, thrombogenesis, the activity of osteoblasts, and the level of ALP in a bone-to-implant interface through a pH-buffering effect. Further studies will be necessary to investigate SA + VUV + BS with respect to its safety and effectiveness in clinical settings. Randomized controlled trials should also be followed to confirm its feasibility in various clinical conditions, such as implant placement immediately after tooth extraction or with simultaneous bone augmentation.

Author Contributions: Conceptualization, C.-J.P. and H.-K.P.; methodology, I.-S.J. and J.-D.S.; software, A.M.K. and H.-K.P.; validation, C.-J.P., K.-G.H., and H.-K.P.; formal analysis, J.H.L., M.T., K.-G.H., and A.M.K.; investigation, I.-S.J. and J.-D.S.; resources, M.T., K.-G.H., and J.H.L.; data curation, H.C., G.-J.C., and C.K.; writing—original draft preparation, C.-J.P. and J.H.L.; writing—review and editing, M.T., H.C., and S.H.J.; visualization, G.-J.C., C.K., and S.H.J.; supervision, H.-K.P. All authors have read and agreed to the published version of the manuscript.

Funding: This research was supported by the research fund of Medicine-Engineering-Bio (MEB) Global Center for Developmental Disorders, Hanyang University (HY-2020-000-0000-2809).

Conflicts of Interest: The authors declare no conflict of interest.

References

1. Özcan, M.; Hämmerle, C. Titanium as a reconstruction and implant material in dentistry: Advantages and pitfalls. *Materials* **2012**, *5*, 1528–1545. [CrossRef]
2. Ehrenfest, D.M.D.; Coelho, P.G.; Kang, B.S.; Sul, Y.T.; Albrektsson, T. Classification of osseointegrated implant surfaces: Materials, chemistry and topography. *Trends Biotechnol.* **2010**, *28*, 198–206. [CrossRef]
3. Milošev, I.; Metikoš-Huković, M.; Strehblow, H.H. Passive film on orthopedic TiAlV alloy formed in physiological solution investigated by X-ray photoelectron spectroscopy. *Biomaterials* **2000**, *21*, 2103–2113. [CrossRef]
4. Lee, J.H.; Ogawa, T. The biological aging of titanium implants. *Implant Dent.* **2012**, *21*, 415–421. [CrossRef]
5. Hori, N.; Att, W.; Ueno, T.; Sato, N.; Yamada, M.; Saruwatari, L.; Suzuki, T.; Ogawa, T. Age-dependent degradation of the protein adsorption capacity of titanium. *J. Dent. Res.* **2009**, *88*, 663–667. [CrossRef]
6. Hori, N.; Ueno, T.; Suzuki, T.; Iwasa, F.; Yamada, M.; Att, W.; Okada, S.; Ohno, A.; Aita, H.; Kimoto, K. Ultraviolet light treatment for the restoration of age-related degradation of titanium bioactivity. *Int. J. Oral Maxillofac. Implant.* **2010**, *25*, 49–62.
7. Ogawa, T. Ultraviolet photofunctionalization of titanium implants. *Int. J. Oral Maxillofac. Implant.* **2014**, *29*, e95–e102. [CrossRef] [PubMed]
8. Rosales-Leal, J.; Rodríguez-Valverde, M.; Mazzaglia, G.; Ramón-Torregrosa, P.; Díaz-Rodríguez, L.; García-Martínez, O.; Vallecillo-Capilla, M.; Ruiz, C.; Cabrerizo-Vílchez, M. Effect of roughness, wettability and morphology of engineered titanium surfaces on osteoblast-like cell adhesion. *Colloids Surf. Physicochem. Eng. Aspects* **2010**, *365*, 222–229. [CrossRef]
9. Cicciù, M.; Fiorillo, L.; Herford, A.S.; Crimi, S.; Bianchi, A.; D'Amico, C.; Laino, L.; Cervino, G. Bioactive titanium surfaces: Interactions of eukaryotic and prokaryotic cells of nano devices applied to dental practice. *Biomedicines* **2019**, *7*, 12. [CrossRef]
10. Li, D.; Ferguson, S.J.; Beutler, T.; Cochran, D.L.; Sittig, C.; Hirt, H.P.; Buser, D. Biomechanical comparison of the sandblasted and acid-etched and the machined and acid-etched titanium surface for dental implants. *J. Biomed. Mater. Res.* **2002**, *60*, 325–332. [CrossRef]
11. Kaysinger, K.K.; Ramp, W.K. Extracellular pH modulates the activity of cultured human osteoblasts. *J. Cell. Biochem.* **1998**, *68*, 83–89. [CrossRef]
12. Marumo, M.; Suehiro, A.; Kakishita, E.; Groschner, K.; Wakabayashi, I. Extracellular pH affects platelet aggregation associated with modulation of store-operated Ca^{2+} entry. *Thromb. Res.* **2001**, *104*, 353–360. [CrossRef]
13. Hong, J.; Kurt, S.; Thor, A. A hydrophilic dental implant surface exhibit thrombogenic properties in vitro. *Clin. Implant Dent. Relat. Res.* **2013**, *15*, 105–112. [CrossRef]
14. Di Iorio, D.; Traini, T.; Degidi, M.; Caputi, S.; Neugebauer, J.; Piattelli, A. Quantitative evaluation of the fibrin clot extension on different implant surfaces: An in vitro study. *J. Biomed. Mater. Res.* **2005**, *74*, 636–642. [CrossRef]
15. Pae, H.C.; Kim, S.K.; Park, J.Y.; Song, Y.W.; Cha, J.K.; Paik, J.W.; Choi, S.H. Bioactive characteristics of an implant surface coated with a pH buffering agent: An in vitro study. *J. Periodontal Implant. Sci.* **2019**, *49*, 366–381. [CrossRef]
16. Cho, Y.S.; Hwang, K.G.; Jun, S.H.; Tallarico, M.; Kwon, A.M.; Park, C.J. Radiologic comparative analysis between saline and platelet-rich fibrin filling after hydraulic transcrestal sinus lifting without adjunctive bone graft: A randomized controlled trial. *Clin. Oral Implant. Res.* **2020**. [CrossRef] [PubMed]

17. Att, W.; Hori, N.; Iwasa, F.; Yamada, M.; Ueno, T.; Ogawa, T. The effect of UV-photofunctionalization on the time-related bioactivity of titanium and chromium–cobalt alloys. *Biomaterials* **2009**, *30*, 4268–4276. [CrossRef]
18. Shie, J.L.; Lee, C.H.; Chiou, C.S.; Chang, C.T.; Chang, C.C.; Chang, C.Y. Photodegradation kinetics of formaldehyde using light sources of UVA, UVC and UVLED in the presence of composed silver titanium oxide photocatalyst. *J. Hazard. Mater.* **2008**, *155*, 164–172. [CrossRef]
19. McGivney, E.; Carlsson, M.; Gustafsson, J.P.; Gorokhova, E. Effects of UV-C and Vacuum-UV TiO_2 advanced oxidation processes on the acute mortality of microalgae. *Photochem. Photobiol.* **2015**, *91*, 1142–1149. [CrossRef]
20. Westall, J.; Hohl, H. A comparison of electrostatic models for the oxide solution interface. *Adv. Colloid Interface Sci.* **1980**, *12*, 265–294. [CrossRef]
21. Tang, L.; Thevenot, P.; Hu, W. Surface chemistry influences implant biocompatibility. *Curr. Top. Med. Chem.* **2008**, *8*, 270–280. [CrossRef]
22. Coelho, P.G.; Granjeiro, J.M.; Romanos, G.E.; Suzuki, M.; Silva, N.R.; Cardaropoli, G.; Thompson, V.P.; Lemons, J.E. Basic research methods and current trends of dental implant surfaces. *J. Biomed. Mater. Res.* **2009**, *88*, 579–596. [CrossRef]
23. Puleo, D.; Nanci, A. Understanding and controlling the bone–implant interface. *Biomaterials* **1999**, *20*, 2311–2321. [CrossRef]
24. Morra, M.; Cassinelli, C.; Cascardo, G.; Mazzucco, L.; Borzini, P.; Fini, M.; Giavaresi, G.; Giardino, R. Collagen I-coated titanium surfaces: Mesenchymal cell adhesion and in vivo evaluation in trabecular bone implants. *J. Biomed. Mater. Res.* **2006**, *78*, 449–458. [CrossRef] [PubMed]
25. Morra, M. Biochemical modification of titanium surfaces: Peptides and ECM proteins. *Eur. Cell. Mater.* **2006**, *12*, 15. [CrossRef]
26. Makowiecki, A.; Hadzik, J.; Błaszczyszyn, A.; Gedrange, T.; Dominiak, M. An evaluation of superhydrophilic surfaces of dental implants-a systematic review and meta-analysis. *BMC Oral Health* **2019**, *19*, 79. [CrossRef]
27. Khandelwal, N.; Oates, T.W.; Vargas, A.; Alexander, P.P.; Schoolfield, J.D.; Alex McMahan, C. Conventional SLA and chemically modified SLA implants in patients with poorly controlled type 2 diabetes mellitus—A randomized controlled trial. *Clin. Oral Implant. Res.* **2013**, *24*, 13–19. [CrossRef]
28. Kokovic, V.; Jung, R.; Feloutzis, A.; Todorovic, V.S.; Jurisic, M.; Hämmerle, C.H. Immediate vs. early loading of SLA implants in the posterior mandible: 5-year results of randomized controlled clinical trial. *Clin. Oral Implant. Res.* **2014**, *25*, e114–e119. [CrossRef]
29. Cesaretti, G.; Botticelli, D.; Renzi, A.; Rossi, M.; Rossi, R.; Lang, N.P. Radiographic evaluation of immediately loaded implants supporting 2–3 units fixed bridges in the posterior maxilla: A 3-year follow-up prospective randomized controlled multicenter clinical study. *Clin. Oral Implant. Res.* **2016**, *27*, 399–405. [CrossRef]
30. Buser, D.; Broggini, N.; Wieland, M.; Schenk, R.; Denzer, A.; Cochran, D.; Hoffmann, B.; Lussi, A.; Steinemann, S. Enhanced bone apposition to a chemically modified SLA titanium surface. *J. Dent. Res.* **2004**, *83*, 529–533. [CrossRef]
31. Lang, N.P.; Salvi, G.E.; Huynh-Ba, G.; Ivanovski, S.; Donos, N.; Bosshardt, D.D. Early osseointegration to hydrophilic and hydrophobic implant surfaces in humans. *Clin. Oral Implant. Res.* **2011**, *22*, 349–356. [CrossRef] [PubMed]
32. Gittens, R.A.; Scheideler, L.; Rupp, F.; Hyzy, S.L.; Geis-Gerstorfer, J.; Schwartz, Z.; Boyan, B.D. A review on the wettability of dental implant surfaces II: Biological and clinical aspects. *Acta Biomater.* **2014**, *10*, 2907–2918. [CrossRef]
33. Shiu, H.T.; Goss, B.; Lutton, C.; Crawford, R.; Xiao, Y. Formation of blood clot on biomaterial implants influences bone healing. *Tissue Eng. Part B Rev.* **2014**, *20*, 697–712. [CrossRef]
34. Yang, J.; Zhou, Y.; Wei, F.; Xiao, Y. Blood clot formed on rough titanium surface induces early cell recruitment. *Clin. Oral Implant. Res.* **2016**, *27*, 1031–1038. [CrossRef]
35. Gassling, V.; Hedderich, J.; Açil, Y.; Purcz, N.; Wiltfang, J.; Douglas, T. Comparison of platelet rich fibrin and collagen as osteoblast-seeded scaffolds for bone tissue engineering applications. *Clin. Oral Implant. Res.* **2013**, *24*, 320–328. [CrossRef]

36. Naik, B.; Karunakar, P.; Jayadev, M.; Marshal, V.R. Role of platelet rich fibrin in wound healing: A critical review. *J. Conserv. Dent.* **2013**, *16*, 284. [CrossRef]
37. Beretta, M.; Poli, P.P.; Pieriboni, S.; Tansella, S.; Manfredini, M.; Cicciù, M.; Maiorana, C. Peri-implant soft tissue conditioning by means of customized healing abutment: A randomized controlled clinical trial. *Materials* **2019**, *12*, 3041. [CrossRef]
38. Kohn, D.H.; Sarmadi, M.; Helman, J.I.; Krebsbach, P.H. Effects of pH on human bone marrow stromal cells in vitro: Implications for tissue engineering of bone. *J. Biomed. Mater. Res.* **2002**, *60*, 292–299. [CrossRef]

Publisher's Note: MDPI stays neutral with regard to jurisdictional claims in published maps and institutional affiliations.

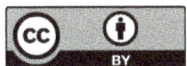 © 2020 by the authors. Licensee MDPI, Basel, Switzerland. This article is an open access article distributed under the terms and conditions of the Creative Commons Attribution (CC BY) license (http://creativecommons.org/licenses/by/4.0/).

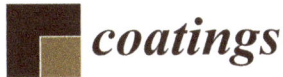

Article

The Use of Autogenous Bone Mixed with a Biphasic Calcium Phosphate in a Maxillary Sinus Floor Elevation Procedure with a 6-Month Healing Time: A Clinical, Radiological, Histological and Histomorphometric Evaluation

Wilhelmus F. Bouwman [1,2], Nathalie Bravenboer [3], Christiaan M. ten Bruggenkate [1,4] and Engelbert A. J. M. Schulten [1,*]

1. Department of Oral and Maxillofacial Surgery/Oral Pathology, Amsterdam UMC and Academic Centre for Dentistry Amsterdam (ACTA), Vrije Universiteit Amsterdam, Amsterdam Movement Sciences, De Boelelaan 1117, 1081 HV Amsterdam, The Netherlands; wbouwman@tergooi.nl (W.F.B.); chris@tenbruggenkate.com (C.M.t.B.)
2. Department of Oral and Maxillofacial Surgery, The Tergooi Hospital, Rijksstraatweg 1, 1261 AN Blaricum, The Netherlands
3. Department of Clinical Chemistry, Amsterdam UMC, Vrije Universiteit Amsterdam, Amsterdam Movement Sciences, De Boelelaan 1117, 1081 HV Amsterdam, The Netherlands; n.bravenboer@amsterdamumc.nl
4. Department of Oral and Maxillofacial Surgery, Alrijne Hospital, Simon Smitweg 1, 2353 GA Leiderdorp, The Netherlands
* Correspondence: eajm.schulten@amsterdamumc.nl; Tel.: +31-(0)20-4441023

Received: 8 April 2020; Accepted: 6 May 2020; Published: 9 May 2020

Abstract: Background: In this study it is evaluated whether autogenous bone mixed with biphasic calcium phosphate (BCP) used in a maxillary sinus floor elevation (MSFE) leads to improved bone formation. Materials and methods: In five patients a unilateral MSFE was performed. Histological and histomorphometric analyses were performed on bone biopsies that were obtained 6 months after MSFE during dental implant surgery. Results: The average vital bone volume was 29.9% of the total biopsy (BV/TV, SD ± 10.1) of which 7.1% was osteoid (OV/BV, SD ± 4.8). The osteoid surface (OS/BS) covered 26.0% (SD ± 13.4) of the bone surface. The BS/TV covered 4.7 mm^2/mm^3 (SD ± 2.3). Compared with previous studies the analyses showed a difference for trabecular thickness (Tb.Th.) and osteoid surface (OS/BS), but not for BV/TV, OV/BV and the number of osteoclasts. Conclusion: MSFE with autogenous bone mixed with BCP shows an amount of newly formed bone that is comparable with the findings from the previously published 6-month study with pure BCP. However, a better distribution of the new bone over the entire biopsy was observed.

Keywords: bone substitute; sinus floor augmentation; maxillary tuberosity

1. Introduction

Lack of vertical bone height in the posterior maxilla limits standard dental implant placement. In order to increase the vertical dimension in the posterior maxilla, a maxillary sinus floor elevation (MSFE) with graft material can be performed. [1,2] MSFE is a predictable preimplant surgical procedure with a high survival rate of the dental implants, exceeding 93.8% [3]. Pjetursson systematically reviewed the success of dental implants placed in combination with MSFE, and reported an implant survival rate after 3 years up to 98.3%, using rough surface dental implants, related to non-augmented jawbone [4].

Due to its osteoinductive, osteoconductive and osteogenic properties autogenous bone is still considered the golden standard as graft material [5–12]. This osteogenic capacity of autogenous bone grafts may be attributed to the presence of bone morphogenic proteins, attracting osteogenic cells from the adjacent tissues, thus mobilizing other growth factors essential for bone regeneration [4].

Bone grafts can be obtained either intraorally or extraorally. Harvesting these bone grafts has drawbacks, such as an extended operating time, donor site morbidity, hospitalization, unpredictable resorption rate of the bone grafts [9,13–15] and sensory disturbances [5,16,17]. Different types of bone substitutes have been developed to overcome these drawbacks (e.g., allograft, xenograft, alloplast and mixtures of different materials) [18,19]. The comparison of bone grafts from different origins has been the subject of study extensively. Meta-analyses have confirmed the superiority of autogenous bone grafts over allografts, xenografts and synthetic bone grafts with respect to new bone formation [20–22]. Ideally, such a bone substitute should be biomechanically stable, capable of degradation within an appropriate time frame, exhibiting osteoconductive, osteogenic and osteoinductive properties, biologically safe, low patient morbidity, volume stable, easy available on the market with low production costs and providing a favorable environment for the entry of blood vessels and bone-forming cells [23–26]. For cranio-maxillofacial purposes, autografts (due to the drawbacks) play a minor role today. In terms of costs and benefits, allografts were the most commonly used bone graft in the United States and xenografts were the most commonly used grafts in Europe [27]. Allografts are tissue grafts from a donor of the same species as the recipient, but not genetically identical, with a risk of immune responses, infection transmission and are known to have high failure rates with long-term use. Additionally, many osteoinductive properties are lost during the manufacturing of allografts [21,28–30]. In Europe, the use of allografts is often abandoned in clinical practice, advised by the Medical Device Regulation [31].

Xenografts are usually of porcine or bovine origin. The use of xenografts involves a number of risks and complications, e.g., disease transmission (Creutzfeldt-Jakob disease), immune responses, foreign body response and chronic inflammation. The production process can lead to a lack of viable cells and reduced osteoinductive properties [32]. For cranio-maxillofacial applications, bovine xenografts are allowed for safe use without reports of transmissible spongiform encephalopathies (TSE) and bovine spongiform encephalopathy (BSE) risk [27,33,34].

Alloplastic (synthetic) grafts are currently most commonly used for their osteoconduction, hardness and acceptability by bone. Most alloplasts consist of hydroxyapatite, a naturally occurring ceramic that is also the primary mineral of bone, or other calcium phosphate compounds, such as β–tricalcium phosphate (β–TCP). Calcium phosphates, like hydroxyapatite (HA), β–tricalcium phosphate (β–TCP) or biphasic calcium phosphate (BCP), a mixture of HA and β-TCP, are osteoconductive, biocompatible and simulate the chemical composition of natural bone. Calcium phosphates do not induce a sustained foreign body response or toxic reaction [35–37]. Hydroxyapatite is, at a physiological pH, the least dissolvable of the naturally occurring calcium phosphates, making it relatively resistant to resorption and suitable for clinical use [9,38–40]. β-TCP does not have osteoinductive properties and resorbs rather quickly, but not necessarily at the same rate as the formation of new bone [11,12,41–44].

In previous studies a mixture of 60% HA and 40% β-TCP (BCP) as graft material in an MSFE procedure demonstrated sufficient bone (re)generation after 6 months for placement of dental implants, although remnants of BCP could still be observed, indicating that the process of bone substitution was not yet completed [12,45]. After 9- and 12-months healing time, a high bone formation was still observed and remnants of BCP particles could still be detected [46]. A significant lower total bone volume is found for each biomaterial or combination of different graft materials compared to autogenous bone [11,47].

This study was based on the use of an autogenous bone graft, harvested from the maxillary tuberosity, in an MSFE procedure, as the golden standard [10]. Though, if autogenous bone graft volume is insufficient, a bone substitute can be supplemented to achieve sufficient graft volume for completion of the MFSE procedure, thereby avoiding a second surgical intervention and minimizing donor site morbidity. Referring to previous studies on the use of BCP's only [12,46], it would be interesting to further study the use of a mixture of autogenous bone and Straumann® Bone Ceramic (SBC), a BCP (Straumann Holding AG, Basel, Switzerland).

Therefore, the purpose of this study was to determine whether a mixture of autogenous bone and BCP in an MSFE procedure leads to an improved bone formation compared to an MSFE with pure BCP and ideally a total remission of BCP remnants in the entire augmented MSFE area, eventually leading to a sufficient bone structure, qualitatively and quantitatively, for dental implant placement. Five subsequent patients were evaluated clinically, radiologically, histologically and histomorphometrically after a 6-month healing period. The results were compared with the results of the previously reported studies with pure BCP (no autogenous bone added), after 6-, 9- and 12-month healing time, which were conducted according to the same study protocol [12,46].

2. Materials and Methods

2.1. Study Population

Five subsequent, healthy patients (3 males and 2 females), with a partially edentulous posterior maxilla with vertical dimensions of less than 8 mm but preferably more than 4 mm, requiring dental implants for dental rehabilitation, were included in this study and underwent a unilateral MSFE procedure 6 months before the dental implants were placed. The average age was 61 years (range: 51–70).

The study was performed in accordance with the principles of the Declaration of Helsinki. Since the study involved a Conformité Européenne (CE)-marked device (biphasic calcium phosphate) being used for its intended purpose (use as carrier material for bone augmentation in sinus floor elevation procedures) and the harvested material is regarded as surgical waste, no specific regulatory approval from a medical ethical committee was required. Patients provided written consent before the study-related MSFE and dental implant procedures were undertaken. Biopsies were retrieved during dental implant surgery, with trephine drills, implicating the tissue in the hollow drill is considered surgical waste and no extra inconvenience to the patient.

2.2. Maxillary Sinus Floor Elevation Procedure

A unilateral two-stage MSFE was performed as described by Tatum [2] and similar to the previously reported 6-month and 9–12-month studies with pure BCP [12,46]. MSFE surgery was performed under local anesthesia. All patients took amoxicillin 500 mg orally, 4 times daily during 7 days, starting one day preoperatively. Oral hygiene was performed with 0.12% chlorhexidine-digluconate 3 times daily for two weeks. The autogenous bone graft was harvested from the maxillary tuberosity at the implant site with mallet and chisel and grinded in small pieces. Before filling the created area at the sinus bottom, the bone graft was mixed in equal proportions with BCP granules (60% HA and 40% β–TCP, Straumann® Bone Ceramic, Straumann Holding AG, Basel, Switzerland). No collagen membrane was placed to cover the lateral window [48] (Figure 1A–E).

2.3. Dental Implant Surgery and Biopsy Retrieval

The dental implants were placed six months after the MSFE procedure. Implant osteotomies were made and biopsies were obtained from the previously grafted area at the planned dental implant positions, using trephine drills with an external diameter of 3.5 mm and internal diameter of 2.5 mm (Straumann® trephine drill) with copious irrigation of sterile saline. In the five patients 11 standard plus, regular neck, soft tissue level Straumann® SLA dental implants with a diameter of 4.1 mm and a length of 10 or 12 mm were placed. (Figure 1F). The dental implants were left to integrate in a non-submerged unloaded fashion. A panoramic radiograph was taken immediately after dental implantation to allow postoperative radiological evaluation. After 10–14 days the Gore-Tex® (W.L.

Gore and Associates, Newark, DE, USA) sutures were removed and, if needed, provisional prosthetics were adapted to the new situation. Loading of the dental implants was prohibited for three months. After osseointegration of the implants, a restorative dentist fabricated and placed the superstructures.

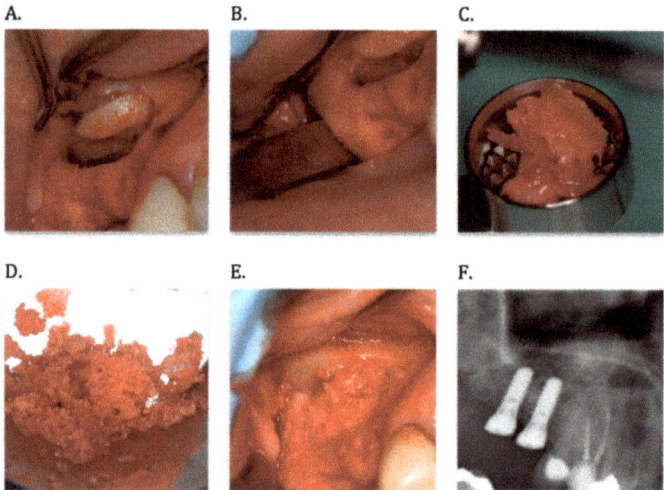

Figure 1. Maxillary sinus floor elevation (MSFE) procedure using a mixture of autogenous bone from the maxillary tuberosity and a biphasic calcium phosphate (BCP). (**A**) The preparation of the top hinge door in the lateral window of the right maxillary sinus. (**B**) Harvesting of an autogenous bone graft from the maxillary tuberosity with a chisel at the same surgical side and during the same procedure. (**C**) The harvested bone graft is grinded in smaller pieces by means of a bone mill. (**D**) The milled bone graft is mixed with a biphasic calcium phosphate (Straumann® Bone Ceramic 60:40). (**E**) Area between the lifted lid and the maxillary sinus floor is filled with the mixed bone graft. (**F**) Radiograph taken directly after the insertion of two Straumann® SLA dental implants in the augmented right posterior maxilla (6 months after MSFE).

2.4. Clinical Evaluation

One experienced oral and maxillofacial surgeon (C.M.T.B.) assessed clinically all 11 inserted dental implants for good primary stability. At abutment connection the osseointegration was tested with a 35 N cm torque. All placed Straumann® SLA dental implants resisted the applied 35 N cm torque.

2.5. Radiological Evaluation

According to the same study protocol as previously reported [12,46], panoramic radiographs were taken at patient's intake (T0); immediately after the MSFE procedure (T1); immediately after dental implant placement (T2); 1 year after dental implant placement (T3) and 5 years after dental implant placement (T4). On the panoramic radiographs changes in tissue height (mm) of the grafted area were measured at the implant sites on all time points. An average magnification of 1.25 was taken into account to calculate the actual tissue heights.

2.6. Biopsy Processing and Analyses

Bone biopsies were prepared for histology according to previously described procedures [49]. In short, the biopsies were fixed overnight in 4% phosphate-buffered formaldehyde and transferred to alcohol 70% [50]. After dehydration, the bone specimens were embedded without prior decalcification in methyl methacrylate supplemented with 20% dibutylphtalaat and 0.008 g/mL Lucidol. The biopsies were cut into 5 μm longitudinal sections (Polycut S., Leica microtome type sm2500s, Leica, Wetzlar,

Germany). Goldner's trichrome staining was used to evaluate bone mass indices and osteoid surface [51]. Tartrate resistant acid phosphate (TRAP) staining was performed to visualize osteoclasts. Von Kossa staining was performed to visualize mineralized tissue.

2.7. Qualitative Histological Analysis

Qualitative assessment included screening the presence of BCP (Straumann® Bone Ceramic) remnants, clearly visible in the Von Kossa staining and a judgment of the vitality of the bone tissue. Moreover, the tissue was screened for inflammatory infiltrate. Three independent observers detected semi-quantitatively BCP particles and classified the particles into quartiles (<25% of BCP, 25%–50%; of BCP, 50%–75% of BCP and >75% of BCP).

2.8. Quantitative Histomorphometric Analysis

Quantitative measurements were performed semiautomatically using a digitizer and image analysis software (Osteomeasure, Atlanta, GA, USA). Since it was difficult to distinguish the exact border between augmented and native bone, histomorphometric measurements were executed over the total section of the biopsy, including newly formed and native bone. The parameters were measured in consecutive fields of a complete section, in four 150 µm-separated sections throughout the biopsy, covering a total measured area of 60 mm^2. Nomenclature was used according to the American Society for Bone and Mineral Research (ASBMR) nomenclature committee [52].

The biopsy was examined for the following parameters:
Parameters evaluating vital bone mass/bone structure:

- Vital bone volume (BV/TV): percentage of the total section that is vital bone tissue (%).
- Bone surface (BS/TV): BS expressed as a fraction of the total vital bone volume (mm^2/mm^3).
- Thickness of bone trabeculae (Tb.Th; µm).

Parameters evaluating bone turnover:

- Osteoid volume (OV/BV): percentage of the vital bone tissue section that is osteoid (%).
- Osteoid surface (OS/BS): osteoid-covered surfaces expressed as the percentage of the total BS (%), to measure new vital bone formation.
- Osteoid thickness (O.Th; µm)
- Number of osteoclasts (N.Oc/BPM) per mm^2 total area.

2.9. Statistical Analysis

Results are expressed as the mean plus or minus standard deviation. The results of this study were compared to the results of previously reported experiments, which were conducted in our institution in a similar manner by use of a non-parametric Kruskal–Wallis test.

3. Results

3.1. Clinical Evaluation

All five patients responded identical. None of them displayed postoperative infections, neither after the MSFE procedure nor after the placement of dental implants. During the insertion of the dental implants, it was observed that the graft material was well vascularized. Although there was a clear demarcation between the grafted area and the original bone of the alveolar process, there was continuity between the graft and the original bone. Although bone substitute particles could still be recognized in the retrieved tissue specimen, the drill remained stable during implant bed preparation. Clinically, all particles appeared to be well integrated in newly formed tissue. All dental implants osseointegrated well and could be loaded with fixed prostheses three months after implant surgery. There was no loss of dental implants during the 5-year follow-up.

3.2. Radiological Evaluation

The results of the alveolar tissue height measurements on panoramic radiographs in time are shown in Table 1. On average an 8.7 mm (SD ± 1.6) increase in height of the grafted area was accomplished using the mentioned MSFE.

Table 1. Alveolar tissue height measurements on panoramic radiographs (in true mm) in five patients in whom a maxillary sinus floor elevation (MSFE) procedure was performed with a mixture of autogenous bone from the maxillary tuberosity and Straumann® Bone Ceramic (60:40) and 6 months healing time.

Patient (N)	Gender/Age	Implant Site	T0	T1	Increase	T2	T3	T4
1	M/53	15	8.0	16.2	8.2	16.1	16.2	16.0
		16	6.1	14.1	8.0	15.0	15.0	15.0
2	M/70	16	6.8	14.8	8.0	16.0	13.7	15.6
		17	3.6	12.4	8.8	14.0	13.3	12.1
3	M/68	14	5.6	11.5	5.9	12.1	11.3	10.4
		15	4.6	14.1	9.5	14.1	13.0	12.9
		16	4.3	14.1	9.8	14.2	12.7	12.6
4	F/64	15	9.3	17.1	7.8	16.8	14.1	14.0
		16	6.0	14.9	8.9	16.9	15.8	15.7
5	M/51	16	9.0	18.1	9.1	17.6	16.2	NA
		17	5.8	18.0	12.2	16.0	16.7	NA
Mean	61.2	-	6.3	15.0	8.7	15.3	14.4	13.8
SD	-	-	1.9	2.1	1.6	1.6	1.7	1.9

M, male; F, female; age in years at biopsy retrieval; tissue height corrected for magnification (×1.25) on panoramic radiograph; T0: (native bone height) preoperative alveolar bone height; T1: directly after MSFE procedure; T2: immediately after dental implant placement (6 months after MSFE); T3: 1 year after dental implant placement; T4: 5 years after dental implant placement; NA: not available.

The measured tissue height appeared to be stable between 1- and 5-years follow-up (Figure 2). The results of the present study (6-month mixed graft) when compared with the results of our former MSFE procedures with pure BCP, also show a stable gain in tissue height (a total of four studies).

An overview of the results of the present study (6-months mixed graft) and the results of previously reported studies with pure BCP after 6-, 9- and 12 months healing time [12,44] is shown in Table 2. Comparing the results, the gained tissue height appears to be stable in all four studies.

Table 2. Alveolar tissue height measurements on panoramic radiographs (in true mm), overview of the mean values of the 6-month mixed graft group, autogenous bone mixed with Straumann® bone ceramic (60:40), compared to the 6-, 9- and 12-month results with pure Straumann® bone ceramic (60:40), as previously published, in a maxillary sinus floor elevation (MSFE) procedure. Tissue height corrected for magnification (×1.25) on panoramic radiographs.

Patient Group	T0	T1	Increase	T2	T3	T4
6-month mixed	6.3	14.8	8.7	15.3	14.4	13.8
6-month (*)	6.5	15.2	8.7	14.6	13.4	NA
9-month (**)	6.4	13.9	7.5	14.1	13.3	13.2
12-month (**)	4.4	13.8	9.3	13.6	13.4	13.8

T0: (native bone height) preoperative alveolar bone height; T1: directly after MSFE procedure; T2: immediately after dental implant placement; T3: 1 year after dental implant placement; T4: 5 years after dental implant placement; NA: not available. * Study by Frenken et al. (2010) [12]; ** Study by Bouwman et al. (2017) [46].

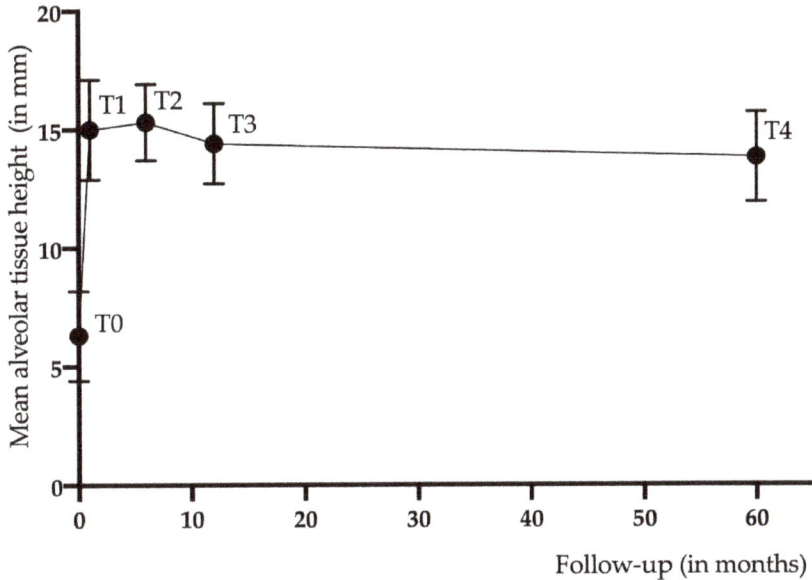

Figure 2. Mean alveolar tissue height (in true mm) over a 5-year period in five patients in whom a maxillary sinus floor elevation procedure was performed with autogenous bone from the maxillary tuberosity and Straumann® bone ceramic (60:40) with 6 months healing period. T0: (native bone height) preoperative alveolar bone height (SD ± 1.9); T1: directly after a maxillary sinus floor elevation (MFSE) procedure (SD ± 2.1); T2: immediately after dental implant placement (6 months after an MSFE; SD ± 1.6); T3: 1 year after dental implant placement (SD ± 1.7); T4: 5 years after dental implant placement (SD ± 1.9).

3.3. Qualitative Histological Evaluation

The histological evaluation in six biopsy specimens was executed on the complete section, comprising native bone, newly formed bone and residual graft material. BCP particles were scattered and detected throughout the entire biopsy from caudal to cranial (Figures 3 and 4a). The BCP particles were surrounded by connective tissue, osteoid islands and newly formed bone. The newly formed bone comprised of both woven and lamellar bone; it appeared as vital bone tissue containing osteoblasts, osteoid covering the border of BCP and osteocytes inside bone lacunae (Figure 4b). No inflammatory cells in the tissue adjacent to the bone substitute particles were found during histological analysis. Bone marrow-like tissue, including blood vessels, was observed in between the bone trabeculae. Fragments of the BCP particles as shown by Von Kossa staining showed in four biopsies <25% of BCP, in one biopsy 25%–50% of BCP and in one biopsy 50%–75% of BCP. The presence of >75% of BCP fragments was not detected.

3.4. Quantitative Histomorphometric Evaluation

Table 3 shows the individual histomorphometric indices. An average vital bone volume of 29.9% (BV/TV) was measured in the complete biopsies (SD ± 10.1) of which 7.1% (OV/BV, SD ± 4.8) was osteoid. The osteoid surface (OS/BS) covered 26.0% (SD ± 13.4) of the bone surface. The BS/TV covered 4.7 mm^2/mm^3 (SD ± 2.3). As can be read from Table 3, Patient #4 had extremely high values for trabecular bone volume (BV/TV and Tb.Th.). This high BV/TV is in accordance with the high T0 value, most likely caused by an oblique section of the cortical maxillary sinus wall (Table 1). A low bone surface (BS/TV: 2.2 mm^2/mm^3) and a high osteoid thickness (O.Th: 481.9 μm) were observed in the bone biopsy of patient #5 (Table 3).

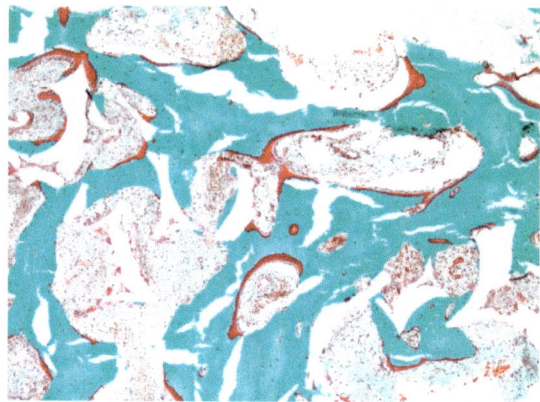

Figure 3. Increased bone formation following the shape of the grafted particles in a maxillary bone biopsy after a maxillary sinus floor elevation procedure from a patient with autogenous bone mixed with Straumann® bone ceramic (60:40) after 6 months healing time, stained with Goldner trichrome staining. No Howship's lacunae could be detected on the characteristic outlines of the calcium phosphate particles. (original magnification ×100).

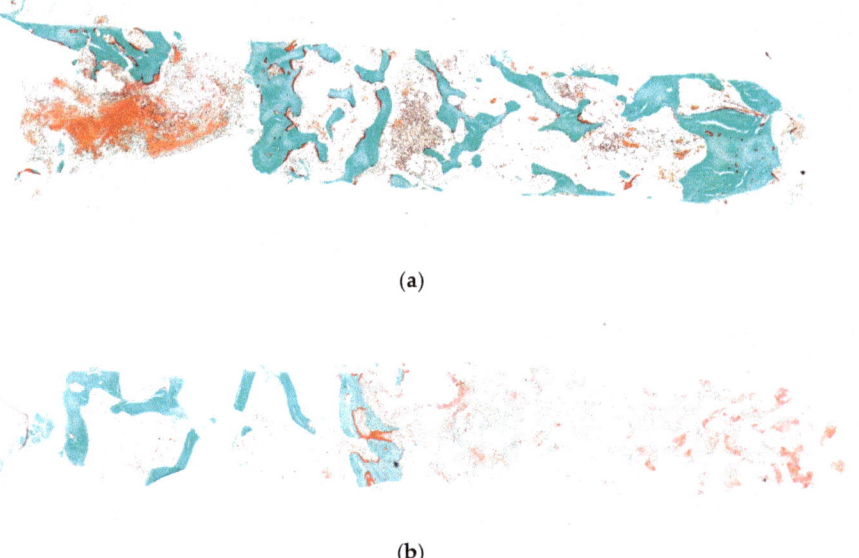

Figure 4. (a) Overview of an example of a bone biopsy from the maxilla of a patient, 6 months after a maxillary sinus floor elevation procedure using a mixture of autogenous bone and Straumann® bone ceramic (60:40), stained with Goldner trichrome staining. Bone is scattered throughout the entire biopsy (original magnification ×10). (b) Overview of a not previously shown bone biopsy from the maxilla of a patient, 6 months after a maxillary sinus floor elevation procedure using pure Straumann® bone ceramic (60:40) as studied by Frenken et al. [12], stained with Goldner trichrome staining. Bone formation at the first 3 mm immediately cranially from the former floor of the maxillary sinus (original magnification ×10).

Table 3. Histomorphometric evaluation of the six biopsies from five patients in whom a maxillary sinus floor elevation (MSFE) procedure was performed with a mixture of autogenous bone from the maxillary tuberosity and Straumann® bone ceramic (60:40) after 6 months healing time.

Patient (N)	Gender/Age	Biopsy Location	BV/TV (%)	BS/TV (mm²/mm³)	Tb.Th (μm)	OV/BV (%)	OS/BS (%)	O.Th (μm)	N.Oc/BPM 1/mm²
1	F/53	16	40.5	2.4	335.8	6.9	38.8	342.2	0.62
2	M/70	16	29.2	6.8	85.5	3.2	11.1	10.7	1.52
3	M/68	14	19.7	6.9	57.5	7.6	17.9	11.6	-
-	-	15	29.3	6.5	91.2	3.5	12.9	11.7	2.54
4	F/64	15	42.4	3.5	290.0	5.1	35.3	97.5	1.91
5	M/51	16	18.3	2.2	163.4	16.3	39.8	481.9	1.58
mean	-	-	29.9	4.7	170.6	7.1	26.0	159.3	1.79
SD	-	-	10.1	2.3	116.6	4.8	13.4	203.5	0.5

M, male; F, female; age in years at biopsy retrieval; BV/TV: vital bone volume/total volume; BS/TV: bone surface/total volume; Tb.Th: trabeculae thickness; OV/BV: osteoid volume/vital bone volume; OS/BS: osteoid surface/bone surface; O.Th: osteoid thickness; N.Oc/BPM: number of osteoclasts per bone perimeter.

Table 3 shows the individual histomorphometric indices. An average vital bone volume of 29.9% (BV/TV) was measured in the complete biopsies (SD ± 10.1) of which 7.1% (OV/BV, SD ± 4.8) was osteoid. The osteoid surface (OS/BS) covered 26.0% (SD ± 13.4) of the bone surface. The BS/TV covered 4.7 mm²/mm³ (SD ± 2.3). As can be read from Table 3, Patient #4 had extremely high values for trabecular bone volume (BV/TV and Tb.Th.). This high BV/TV is in accordance with the high T0 value, most likely caused by an oblique section of the cortical maxillary sinus wall (Table 1). A low bone surface (BS/TV: 2.2 mm²/mm³) and a high osteoid thickness (O.Th: 481.9 μm) were observed in the bone biopsy of patient #5 (Table 3).

An overview of the histomorphometric findings from the present study (6-months mixed graft) and previously reported studies with pure BCP after 6-, 9- and 12 months healing time is shown in Table 4. A non-parametric Kruskal–Wallis test showed significant differences between OS/BS ($p = 0.0233$) and Tb.Th. ($p = 0.0244$). Other tested histomorphometric indices (BV/TV, OV/BV, and N.Oc/BPM) were not different.

Table 4. Histomorphometric evaluation of the total section: overview of the mean values of the 6-month mixed graft group (autogenous bone mixed with Straumann® bone ceramic (60:40)) compared to the 6-, 9- and 12-month results with pure Straumann® bone ceramic (60:40), as previously published, in a maxillary sinus floor elevation procedure.

Patient Group	BV/TV (%)	SD ±	BS/TV (mm²/mm³)	SD ±	Tb.Th (μm)	SD ±	OV/BV (%)	SD ±	OS/BS (%)	SD ±	O.Th (μm)	SD ±	N.Oc/BPM 1/mm²	SD ±
6-month mixed	29.9	10.1	4.7	2.3	170.6	116.6	7.1	4.8	26.0	13.4	159.3	203.5	1.79	0.5
6-month (*)	27.3	4.9	4.5	1.1	132.1	38.4	7.5	4.3	41.3	28.5	13.3	4.7	1.1	1.3
9-month (**)	35.2	9.5	4.2	1.9	224.7	150.0	8.8	3.8	42.4	12.1	93.9	135.8	1.8	1.1
12-month (**)	28.2	3.2	8.3	1.3	66.7	5.4	3.4	2.5	8.2	5.3	13.6	1.0	***	-

BV/TV: vital bone volume/total volume; BS/TV: bone surface/total volume; Tb.Th: trabeculae thickness; OV/BV: osteoid volume/vital bone volume; OS/BS: osteoid surface/bone surface; O.Th: osteoid thickness; N.Oc/BPM: number of osteoclasts per bone perimeter. * Study by Frenken et al. (2010) [12]; ** Study by Bouwman et al. (2017) [46]; *** N.Oc/BPM not measured as an insignificant number of osteoclasts were available.

4. Discussion

Addition of Straumann® bone ceramic (60:40; BCP) to autogenous bone did not seem to improve the outcome after 6 months healing time compared to the use of pure BCP in an MSFE, as demonstrated by histomorphometric analyses in the five patients included in the present study. Histomorphometric indices show a high variability, which in most cases can be explained individually. For instance, an oblique section of the cortical maxillary sinus wall could explain, to some extent, the variability mentioned. Compared to autogenous bone, for each biomaterial or combination of graft materials in a maxillary sinus floor elevation (MSFE) procedure a significant lower BV/TV was found (reference value 41% for autogenous bone) [53]. The autogenous bone graft, in the present study was harvested from the maxillary tuberosity, at the same side as the MSFE procedure was performed, implicating no extra or at least far less morbidity for the patient. However, the disadvantages of a second surgical procedure of harvesting a bone graft should also be taken into account. This disadvantage remains in the situation of a mixed graft, consisting of autogenous bone and a bone substitute.

Since the procedures in this study were similar to the procedures in the previously reported studies using pure BCP as a bone substitute in an MFSE procedure [12,32], it was possible to compare the histomorphometric findings. This analysis showed a difference for trabecular thickness (Tb.Th.) and osteoid surface (OS/BS) but not for the other parameters (BV/TV, OV/BV, and N.Oc/BPM). The osteoid surface suggested a gradual decrease over healing time for pure BCP while the 6-months mixed graft group did not fit in this pattern, which suggests a different healing pattern. Surprisingly, the presence of autogenous bone in the graft does not seem to result in a higher bone volume at 6-months healing time. According to Klijn et al. [9], a healing time of 6 months may not show the ultimate favorable effect in bone regeneration procedures.

In this study, no dental implants were lost during the 5-year follow-up. A minimum native bone height of 4 mm was chosen as a prerequisite to ensure primary stability and high survival rates of the dental implants [12,46] after an MSFE procedure with a bone substitute, regardless of the type of graft used. Klijn et al. indicated that the measured bone volumes are higher in the first stage of healing (first 4.5 months) and in the later stages of healing after 9 months, which indicates that our study design of 6 months healing time does not entirely demonstrate the advantage of adding a bone substitute to autogenous bone. It should, however, be stressed that an MSFE procedure using pure autogenous bone provides a higher vital bone volume after 6 months if a block graft is used compared to a particulate graft or a mixed graft of autogenous bone with a bone substitute [9]. This is also confirmed by meta-analyses on histomorphometric outcome of bone substitutes and autogenous bone grafts in various combinations. Altogether, autogenous bone (and if needed a mixture of autogenous bone with BCP) is superior in terms of the amount of the newly formed bone.

The low number of patients ($n = 5$) in this study was considered a limitation since quantitative histomorphometric data may be less reliable. Indeed, the histomorphometric indices do not always show a clear difference between pure BCP and autogenous bone mixed with BCP. However, qualitative assessment, in contrast, demonstrated consistently a different distribution of bone throughout all biopsies. In the 6-months mixed graft group bone matrix was scattered throughout the entire biopsy with a slightly less dense trabecular pattern in the centers of the grafted area, while in the 6-months pure BCP group a concentration of bone formation at the first 3 mm immediately cranially from the former floor of the maxillary sinus and less bone in the center of the graft was seen. This might be beneficial for bone-to-implant contact (BIC).

Dental implants are endosseous implants, which implicates that the implant should be anchored in and surrounded by vital bone for a stable result with a high (and long lasting) survival rate. In that respect the presence of vital bone over a larger area in grafted sites is important for the longevity of the dental implants to be inserted later. In this study, a minimal native bone height of 4 mm was required to achieve a good primary stability after the MSFE procedure. Using 100% autogenous bone in the MSFE procedure could shorten the healing time to 4 months and would result in a better BIC. If no or not enough autogenous bone is available, alternatively a bone substitute could be added in the MSFE procedure to achieve a good BIC. However, longer healing times (6-, 9- or 12 months studies) should be respected. In our previous studies with pure BCP the optimal healing time seemed to be 9 months, based on the BV/TV, Tb.Th. and O.Th. observed [45]. In cases with less than 4 mm native bone height, an autogenous bone graft is preferably used in an MSFE procedure. If the availability of autogenous bone is limited, it may be considered to use a mixture of autogenous bone and bone substitute to achieve on the one hand a larger graft volume and on the other hand a larger bone volume, that approximates the bone volume in case a full autogenous bone graft is used. The newly formed bone in the present mixed graft study was observed throughout the entire biopsy, suggesting a large

BIC after 6 months. However, the consequences of these findings for dental implant survival still have to be unraveled.

5. Conclusions

Based on clinical, radiological, histological and histomorphometric analyses in this study with five patients, the use of an autogenous bone graft mixed with a biphasic calcium phosphate (BCP) in a maxillary sinus floor elevation procedure does not result in a higher bone formation, compared with the results of previously reported studies with pure BCP. However, a better distribution of new bone was seen throughout the entire augmented area, which might eventually improve the bone-to-implant contact.

Author Contributions: Conceptualization, W.F.B., C.M.t.B., and E.A.J.M.S.; methodology, W.F.B., N.B., C.M.t.B., and E.A.J.M.S.; validation, W.F.B., N.B., C.M.t.B., and E.A.J.M.S.; formal analysis, W.F.B. and N.B.; investigation, W.F.B., N.B., and C.M.t.B.; data curation, W.F.B.; writing—original draft preparation, W.F.B.; writing—review and editing, W.F.B., N.B., C.M.t.B., and E.A.J.M.S.; visualization, W.F.B.; supervision, E.A.J.M.S. All authors have read and agreed to the published version of the manuscript.

Funding: This research received no external funding.

Acknowledgments: We are grateful to H. van Essen for technical assistance.

Conflicts of Interest: The authors declare no conflict of interest.

Abbreviations

ASBMR	American Society for Bone and Mineral Research
BCP	biphasic calcium phosphate
BIC	bone-to-implant contact
BPM	bone perimeter
BV/TV	bone volume/total volume
BS/TV	bone surface/total volume
C.M.T.B.	Christiaan M. ten Bruggenkate
CE	Conformité Européenne
HA	hydroxyapatite
MSFE	maxillary sinus floor elevation
NA	not available
N.Oc	number of osteoclasts
O.Th	osteoid thickness
OS/BS	osteoid surface/bone surface
OV/BV	osteoid volume/bone volume
SBC	Straumann® Bone Ceramic
Tb.Th	trabecular thickness
TRAP	tartrate resistant acid phosphate
β–TCP	β–tricalcium phosphate

References

1. Boyne, P.J.; James, R.A. Grafting of the maxillary sinus floor with autogenous marrow and bone. *J. Oral Surg.* **1980**, *38*, 613–616. [PubMed]
2. Tatum, H., Jr. Maxillary and sinus implant reconstructions. *Dent Clin. N. Am.* **1986**, *30*, 207–229. [PubMed]
3. Del Fabbro, M.; Rosano, G.; Taschieri, S. Implant survival rates after maxillary sinus augmentation. *Eur. J. Oral Sci.* **2008**, *116*, 497–506. [CrossRef] [PubMed]
4. Pjetursson, B.E.; Tan, W.C.; Zwahlen, M.; Lang, N.P. A systematic review of the success of sinus floor elevation and survival of implants inserted in combination with sinus floor elevation. Part, I.; Lateral approach. *J. Clin. Periodontol.* **2008**, *35*, 216–240. [CrossRef]
5. Burchardt, H. The biology of bone graft repair. *Clin. Orthop. Relat. Res.* **1983**, *174*, 28–42. [CrossRef]

6. Jensen, O.T.; Shulman, L.B.; Block, M.S.; Iacono, V.J. Report of the Sinus Consensus Conference of 1996. *Int. J. Oral Maxillofac. Implant.* **1998**, *13*, 11–45.
7. Tong, D.C.; Rioux, K.; Drangsholt, M.; Beirne, O.R. A review of survival rates for implants placed in grafted maxillary sinuses using meta-analysis. *Int. J. Oral Maxillofac. Implant.* **1998**, *13*, 175–182.
8. Van den Bergh, J.P.; ten Bruggenkate, C.M.; Krekeler, G.; Tuinzing, D.B. Sinus floor elevation and grafting with autogenous iliac crest bone. *Clin. Oral Implant. Res.* **1998**, *9*, 429–435. [CrossRef]
9. Klijn, R.J.; Meijer, G.J.; Bronkhorst, E.M.; Jansen, J.A. A meta-analysis of histomorphometric results and graft healing time of various biomaterials compared to autologous bone used as sinus floor augmentation material in humans. *Tissue Eng. Part B Rev.* **2010**, *16*, 493–507. [CrossRef]
10. Misch, C.M. Autogenous Bone: Is It Still the Gold Standard? *Implant Dent.* **2010**, *19*, 361. [CrossRef]
11. Nkenke, E.; Stelzle, F. Clinical outcomes of sinus floor augmentation for implant placement using autogenous bone or bone substitutes: A systematic review. *Clin. Oral Implant. Res.* **2009**, *20* (Suppl. 4), 124–133. [CrossRef] [PubMed]
12. Frenken, J.W.; Bouwman, W.F.; Bravenboer, N.; Zijderveld, S.A.; Schulten, E.A.J.M. The use of Straumann® Bone Ceramic in a maxillary sinus floor elevation procedure: A clinical radiological histological and histomorphometric evaluation with a 6-month healing period. *Clin. Oral Implant. Res.* **2010**, *21*, 201–208. [CrossRef] [PubMed]
13. Kalk, W.W.; Raghoebar, G.M.; Jansma, J.; Boering, G. Morbidity from iliac crest bone harvesting. *Int. J. Oral Maxillofac. Implant.* **1996**, *54*, 1424–1429. [CrossRef]
14. Raghoebar, G.M.; Louwerse, C.; Kalk, W.W.; Vissink, A. Morbidity of chin bone harvesting. *Clin. Oral Implant. Res.* **2001**, *12*, 503–507. [CrossRef]
15. Zijderveld, S.A.; ten Bruggenkate, C.M.; Van Den Bergh, J.P.; Schulten, E.A.J.M. Fractures of the iliac crest after split-thickness bone grafting for preprosthetic surgery: Report of 3 cases and review of the literature. *J. Oral Maxillofac. Surg.* **2004**, *7*, 781–786. [CrossRef]
16. Beirne, J.C.; Barry, H.J.; Brady, F.A.; Morris, V.B. Donor site morbidity of the anterior iliac crest following cancellous bone harvest. *Int. J. Oral Maxillofac. Implant.* **1996**, *25*, 268–271. [CrossRef]
17. Vermeeren, J.I.J.F.; Wismeijer, D.; Van Waas, M.A.J. One-step reconstruction of the severely resorbed mandible with onlay bone grafts and endosteal implants: A 5-year follow-up. *Int. J. Oral Maxillofac. Implant.* **1996**, *2*, 112–115. [CrossRef]
18. Haugen, H.J.; Lyngstadaas, S.P.; Rossi, F.; Perale, G. Bone grafts: Which is the ideal biomaterial? *J. Clin. Periodontol.* **2019**, *46* (Suppl. 21), 92–102. [CrossRef]
19. Rothermundt, C.; Whelan, J.; Dileo, P.; Strauss, S.; Coleman, J.; Briggs, T.; Seddon, B. What is the role of routine follow-up forlocalised limb soft tissue sarcomas? A retrospective analysis of 174 patients. *Br. J. Cancer* **2014**, *110*, 2420. [CrossRef]
20. Corbella, S.; Taschieri, S.; Weinstein, R.; Del Fabbro, M. Histomorphometric outcomes after lateral sinus floor elevation procedure: A systematic review of the literature and meta-analysis. *Clin. Oral Implant. Res.* **2016**, *27*, 1106–1122. [CrossRef]
21. De Grado, G.F.; Keller, L.; Idoux-Gillet, Y.; Wagner, Q.; Musset, A.M.; Benkirane-Jessel, N.; Offner, D. Bone substitutes: A review of their characteristics, clinical use, and perspectives for large bone defects management. *J. Tissue Eng.* **2018**, *9*. [CrossRef]
22. Papageorgiou, S.N.; Papageorgiou, P.N.; Deschner, J.; Götz, W. Comparative effectiveness of natural and synthetic bone grafts in oral and maxillofacial surgery prior to insertion of dental implants: Systematic review and network meta-analysis of parallel and cluster randomized controlled trials. *J. Dent.* **2016**, *48*, 1–8. [CrossRef] [PubMed]
23. Bose, S.; Roy, M.; Bandyopadhyay, A. Recent advances in bone tissue engineering scaffolds. *Trends Biotechnol.* **2012**, *30*, 546–554. [CrossRef] [PubMed]
24. El-Rashidy, A.A.; Roether, J.A.; Harhaus, L.; Kneser, U.; Boccaccini, A.R. Regenerating bone with bioactive glass scaffolds: A review of in vivo studies in bone defect models. *Acta Biomater.* **2017**, 1–28. [CrossRef]
25. Hutmacher, D.W. *Scaffolds in Tissue Engineering Bone Andcartilage. The Biomaterials: Silver Jubilee Compendium*; Elsevier Science: Oxford, UK, 2006; pp. 175–189.
26. Janicki, P.; Schmidmaier, G. What should be the characteristics of the ideal bone graft substitute? Combining scaffolds with growth factors and/or stem cells. *Injury* **2011**, S77–S81. [CrossRef]

27. Jo, S.H.; Kim, Y.K.; Choi, Y.H. Histological Evaluation of the Healing Process of Various Bone Graft Materials after Engraftment into the Human Body. *Materials* **2018**, *11*, 714. [CrossRef]
28. Delloye, C.; Cornu, O.; Druez, V.; Barbier, O. Bone allografts: What they can offer and what they cannot. *J. ofBone Joint Surg. Br. Vol.* **2007**, *89*, 574–579. [CrossRef]
29. Wheeler, D.L.; Enneking, W.F. Allograft bone decreases in strength in vivo over time. *Clin. Orthop. Relat. Res.* **2005**, 36–42. [CrossRef]
30. Winkler, T.; Sass, F.A.; Duda, G.N.; Schmidt-Bleek, K. A review of biomaterials in bone defect healing, remaining shortcomings and future opportunities for bone tissue engineering THE UNSOLVED CHALLENGE. *Bone Jt. Res.* **2018**, *7*, 232–243. [CrossRef]
31. MDR. Regulation (EU) 2017/745 of The European Parliament and of the Council of 5 April 2017 on Medical devices Retrieved. Available online: http://data.europa.eu/eli/reg/2017/2745/oj (accessed on 5 April 2017).
32. Zimmermann, G.; Moghaddam, A. Allograft bone matrix versus synthetic bone graft substitutes. *Inj. -Int. Care Inj.* **2011**, *42*, S16–S21. [CrossRef]
33. Kim, Y.; Nowzari, H.; Rich, S.K. Risk of prion disease transmission through bovine-derived bone substitutes: A systematic review. *Clin. Implant Dent. Relat. Res.* **2013**, *15*, 645–653. [CrossRef]
34. Yamada, M.; Egusa, H. Current bone substitutes for implant dentistry. *J. Prosthodont. Res.* **2018**, *62*, 152–161. [CrossRef]
35. Nery, E.B.; Lee, K.K.; Czajkowski, S.; Dooner, J.J.; Duggan, M.; Ellinger, R.F.; Henkin, J.M.; Hines, R.; Miller, M.; Olson, J.W.; et al. A Veterans Administration Cooperative Study of biphasic calcium phosphate ceramic in periodontal osseous defects. *J. Periodontol.* **1990**, *61*, 737–744. [CrossRef]
36. Zerbo, I.R.; Bronckers, A.L.; de Lange, G.; Burger, E.H. Localisation of osteogenic and osteoclastic cells in porous beta-tricalcium phosphate particles used for human maxillary sinus floor elevation. *Biomaterials* **2005**, *26*, 1445–1451. [CrossRef] [PubMed]
37. Joosten, U.; Joist, A.; Frebel, T.; Walter, M.; Langer, M. The use of an in situ curing hydroxyapatite cement as an alternative to bone graft following removal of enchondroma of the hand. *J. Hand Surg. Br. Eur. Vol.* **2000**, *25*, 288–291. [CrossRef] [PubMed]
38. Costantino, P.D.; Friedman, C.D.; Jones, K.; Chow, L.C.; Pelzer, H.J.; Sisson, G.A. Hydroxyapatite cement: I. Basic chemistry and histologic properties. *Arch. Otolaryngol. Head Neck Surg.* **1991**, *117*, 384–397. [CrossRef] [PubMed]
39. Costantino, P.D.; Friedman, C.D. Synthetic bone graft substitutes. *Otolaryngol. Clin. N. Am.* **1994**, *27*, 1037–1074.
40. Jensen, S.S.; Aaboe, M.; Pinholt, E.M.; Hjorting-Hansen, E.; Melsen, F.; Ruyter, I.E. Tissue reaction and material characteristics of four bone substitutes. *Int. J. Oral Maxillofac. Implant.* **1996**, *11*, 55–66.
41. Daculsi, G.; Laboux, O.; Malard, O.; Weiss, P. Current state of the art of biphasic calcium phosphate bioceramics. *J. Mater. Sci. Mater. Med.* **2003**, *14*, 195–200. [CrossRef]
42. LeGeros, R.Z.; Lin, S.; Rohanizadeh, R.; Mijares, D.; LeGeros, J.P. Biphasic calcium phosphate bioceramics: Preparation properties and applications. *J. Mater. Sci. Mater. Med.* **2003**, *14*, 201–209. [CrossRef]
43. Schopper, C.; Ziya-Ghazvini, F.; Goriwoda, W.; Moser, D.; Wanschitz, F.; Spassova, E.; Lagogiannis, G.; Auterith, A.; Ewers, R. HA/TCP compounding of a porous CaP biomaterial improves bone formation and scaffold degradation—A long-term histological study. *J. Biomed. Mater. Res. B Appl. Biomater.* **2005**, *74*, 458–467. [CrossRef]
44. Zerbo, I.R.; Zijderveld, S.A.; De Boer, A.; Bronckers, A.L.J.J.; De Lange, G.; ten Bruggenkate, C.M.; Burger, E.H. Histomorphometry of human sinus floor augmentation using a porous beta-tricalcium phosphate: A prospective study. *Clin. Oral Implant. Res.* **2004**, *15*, 724–732. [CrossRef] [PubMed]
45. Groeneveld, E.H.; van den Bergh, J.P.; Holzmann, P.; ten Bruggenkate, C.M.; Tuinzing, D.B.; Burger, E.H. Mineralization processes in demineralized bone matrix grafts in human maxillary sinus floor elevations. *J. Biomed. Mater. Res.* **1999**, *48*, 393–402. [CrossRef]
46. Bouwman, W.F.; Bravenboer, N.; Frenken, J.W.F.H.; ten Bruggenkate, C.M.; Schulten, E.A.J.M. The use of a biphasic calcium phosphate in a maxillary sinus floor elevation procedure: A clinical radiological histological and histomorphometric evaluation with 9- and 12-month healing times. *Int. J. Implant Dent.* **2017**, *3*, 34. [CrossRef] [PubMed]
47. Wheeler, S.L. Sinus augmentation for dental implants: The use of alloplastic materials. *J. Oral Maxillofac. Surg.* **1997**, *55*, 1287–1293. [CrossRef]

48. Schulten, E.A.J.M.; Prins, H.J.; Overman, J.R.; Helder, M.N.; ten Bruggenkate, C.M.; Klein-Nuland, J. A novel approach revealing the effect of collagenous membrane on osteoconduction in maxillary sinus floor elevation with β-tricalcium phosphate. *Eur. Cells Mater.* **2013**, *25*, 215–228. [CrossRef]
49. Oostlander, A.E.; Bravenboer, N.; Sohl, E.; Holzmann, P.J. Dutch Initiative on Crohn and Colitis (ICC). Histomorphometric analysis reveals reduced bone mass and bone formation in patients with quiescent Crohn's disease. *Gastroenterology* **2011**, *140*, 116–123. [CrossRef]
50. Schenk, R.K.; Olah, A.J.; Herrmann, W. Preparation of calcified tissues for light microscopy. In *Methods of Calcified Tissue Preparation*; Dickson, G.R., Ed.; Elsevier Science Publishers: Amsterdam, The Netherlands, 1983; Volume 1, p. 56.
51. Romeis, B. *Trichromfaerbung nach Goldner Mikroskopische Technik*; Urban & Schwarzenberg: Muenchen, Germany, 1989.
52. Dempster, D.W.; Compston, J.E.; Drezner, M.K.; Glorieux, F.H.; Kanis, J.A.; Malluche, H.; Meunier, P.J.; Ott, S.M.; Recker, R.R.; Parfitt, A.M. Standardized nomenclature symbols and units for bone histomorphometry: A 2012 update of the report of the ASBMR Histomorphometry Nomenclature Committee. *J. Bone Miner. Res.* **2012**. [CrossRef]
53. Zijderveld, S.A.; Zerbo, I.R.; Van den Bergh, J.P.A.; Schulten, E.A.J.M.; ten Bruggenkate, C.M. Maxillary Sinus Floor Augmentation Using a β–Tricalcium Phosphate (Cerasorb) Alone Compared to Autogenous Bone Grafts. *Int. J. Oral Maxillofac. Implant.* **2005**, *20*, 432–440.

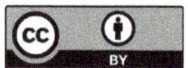

© 2020 by the authors. Licensee MDPI, Basel, Switzerland. This article is an open access article distributed under the terms and conditions of the Creative Commons Attribution (CC BY) license (http://creativecommons.org/licenses/by/4.0/).

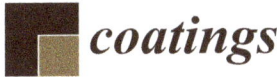

Article

The Effects of Bone Morphogenetic Protein-4 on Cellular Viability, Osteogenic Potential, and Global Gene Expression on Gingiva-Derived Stem Cell Spheroids

Jae-Yong Tae [1,2], Yoon-Hee Park [3], Youngkyung Ko [1,2] and Jun-Beom Park [1,2,*]

1. Department of Medicine, Graduate School, The Catholic University of Korea, Seoul 06591, Korea; taejaeyong@naver.com (J.-Y.T.); ko_y@catholic.ac.kr (Y.K.)
2. Department of Periodontics, College of Medicine, The Catholic University of Korea, Seoul 06591, Korea
3. ebiogen, Seonyu-ro 13-gil, Yeongdeungpo-gu, Seoul 07282, Korea; yhpark@e-biogen.com
* Correspondence: jbassoon@catholic.ac.kr; Tel.: +82-10-4325-2651

Received: 15 September 2020; Accepted: 22 October 2020; Published: 30 October 2020

Abstract: Bone morphogenetic protein-4 (BMP-4) is engaged in the migration ability of mesenchymal stem cells and the transition of mesenchymal stem cells into osteogenic and adipocytic lines. The aim of this study was to evaluate the effects of BMP-4 on the cellular viability, osteogenic differentiation, and genome-wide mRNA levels using three-dimensional cell spheroids composed of stem cells. Stem cell spheroids were formed using concave microwells in the presence of BMP-4 with final concentrations of 0, 2, 6, and 10 ng/mL. Cellular viability was measured qualitatively using a microscope and quantitatively using an assay kit based on water-soluble tetrazolium salt. Osteogenic differentiation was assessed by measuring the level of alkaline phosphatase activity. Global gene expression was assessed using next-generation mRNA sequencing and performing gene ontology and pathway analyses. Spheroids were well-maintained with the addition of BMP-4 up to Day 7. No significant differences were observed in cell viability between each group. There were significantly higher alkaline phosphatase values in the 2 ng/mL BMP-4 groups when compared with the control ($p < 0.05$). A total of 25,737 mRNAs were differentially expressed. Expression of β-catenin (CTNNB1) was increased with higher dosages of BMP-4. The expression of runt-related transcription factor 2 (RUNX2) was increased up to 6 ng/mL. The phosphoinositide-3-kinase–protein kinase B/Akt signaling pathway was associated with the target genes. This study demonstrates that the application of BMP-4 enhanced alkaline phosphatase activity and the expression of CTNNB1 and RUNX2 without affecting cellular viability.

Keywords: bone morphogenetic protein 4; cell differentiation; cellular spheroids; gingiva osteogenesis; stem cells

1. Introduction

Mesenchymal stem cells (MSCs) are multipotent cells that can differentiate into the mesenchymal lineage and easily cultured in vitro [1]. A previous study demonstrated that stem cell spheroids of various sizes could be generated from gingival cells using microwells and that the shape and viability of the spheroids could be maintained [2]. Furthermore, cell spheroids made from gingival cells and osteoblast cells were able to maintain shape, viability, and osteogenic differentiation ability [3]. Stem cell therapy has been of great interest in recent years [4]. A two-dimensional culture has long been applied for the evaluation of viability and functionality of stem cells [3]. In more recent years, three-dimensional cultures have been used by applying various methods including the hanging drop method, bioreactor, capsules, and microwells [5]. Three-dimensional cultures have been reported to mimic the in vivo situation more closely [6]. A three-dimensional culture can be categorized by scaffold-based or scaffold-free application [7]. Three-dimensional spheroids can be made of a variety of cells including stem cells with the scaffold-free technique [8]. Spheroids can be used to obtain an overall enhancement in therapeutic potential by improving survival, stemness, angiogenic properties, and anti-inflammatory effects [9].

Bone morphogenetic proteins (BMPs) are powerful growth factors in the transforming growth factor beta superfamily [10]. More than twenty members with various functions have already been identified in humans, with roles in processes such as skeletal formation, hematopoiesis, and neurogenesis [11]. These BMPs are soluble local-acting signaling proteins that may behave in an endocrine, paracrine, or autocrine manner [12]. BMP-4 may be involved in various functions, including enhancing the migration ability of mesenchymal stem cells and the transition from mesenchymal stem cells into the osteogenic and adipocytic lines [13,14]. BMP-4 may act as an important regulator for proper reproductive tissue development [15]. Moreover, BMP-4 is reported to be involved in postnatal tooth cytodifferentiation [16]. BMP-4 has been suggested as a coating material for titanium implants [17]. To the best of the authors' knowledge, there are no previous studies evaluating the effects of BMP-4 on the cell spheroids composed of gingiva-derived stem cells using microwells. In light of the promising findings in previous studies on BMP-4, the aim of the present study was to evaluate the effects of BMP-4 on cellular viability, osteogenic differentiation, and genome-wide mRNA levels using stem cell spheroids.

2. Materials and Methods

2.1. Formation of Cell Spheroids with Gingiva-Derived Stem Cells

Cell spheroids were made of gingiva-derived mesenchymal stem cells using the concave microwells made of silicone elastomer having 600 µm diameters (H389600, StemFIT 3D; MicroFIT, Seongnam, Korea). The number of cells loaded in each well was 1×10^6. We obtained approval from the Institutional Review Board at Seoul St Mary's Hospital, Seoul, Korea (KC20SISE0695), and informed consent was obtained from the participant. Cell spheroids made were treated with BMP-4 (ProSpec, Ness-Ziona, Israel) at 0, 2, 6, and 10 ng/mL concentrations. The morphological changes in cell spheroids were observed under an inverted microscope (Leica DM IRM, Leica Microsystems, Wetzlar, Germany). The changes in the spheroids' diameter were evaluated on Days 1, 3, 5, and 7. The diameter of the spheroids was determined as described in a previous study [18]. Figure 1 diagrams the overall design of the study.

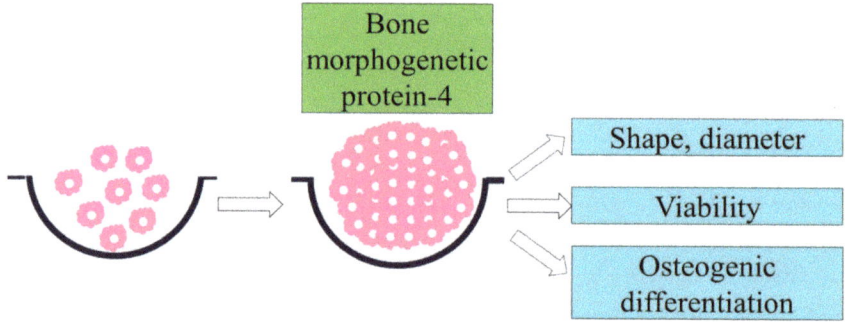

Figure 1. Schematic overview of the present study's design.

2.2. Evaluation of Cellular Viability

Qualitative analysis of the cell spheroids for cellular viability was done using the Live/Dead assay kit (Molecular Probes, Eugene, OR, USA). These spheroids were washed twice with the growth media before calcein acetoxymethyl (Molecular Probes) and ethidium homodimer-1 (Molecular Probes) were added for an incubation period of 30 min at room temperature. Then, the spheroids were evaluated using a fluorescence microscope (Axiovert 200; Zeiss, Oberkochen, Germany) on Days 3 and 7.

Quantitative analysis of cell viability was performed using the cell counting kit-8 (CCK-8; Dojindo, Tokyo, Japan) on Days 1, 3, 5, and 7. WST-8 solution was added to the stem cell spheroids, which were then cultured for 45 min at 37 °C. Absorbance was measured using a microplate reader at 450 nm (BioTek, Winooski, VT, USA).

2.3. Evaluation of Osteogenic Differentiation Using Alkaline Phosphatase Activity Assays

Cell spheroids were grown in osteogenic medium and were collected on Days 1, 3, 5, and 7. A commercially available alkaline phosphatase assay kit (K412-500, BioVision, Inc., Milpitas, CA, USA) was used for the evaluation of osteogenic differentiation. In short, the resultant supernatant was mixed and incubated with p-nitrophenyl phosphate substrate (BioVision, Inc.) for 40 min at room temperature. Absorbance was measured using a microplate reader at 405 nm (BioTek, Winooski, VT, USA).

2.4. Sequencing of mRNA, Gene Ontology, and Pathway Analysis

Construction of a library of RNAs was performed using the SENSE mRNA-Seq Library Prep Kit (Lexogen, Inc., Vienna, Austria). Briefly, 2 μg of total RNA was processed and incubated with oligo-dT magnetic beads, after which other RNAs except mRNA were eliminated with a washing solution. Random hybridization of starter/stopper heterodimers was applied to the poly(A)RNA still bound to the magnetic beads in order to produce libraries. These heterodimers consisted of Illumina-compatible linker sequences. A single-tube reverse transcription and ligation reaction was applied to extend the starter to the next hybridized heterodimer. Then, the newly synthesized cDNA insert was bound with the stopper. The release of the library from the beads was done by second-strand synthesis. The library was amplified afterward and bar codes were introduced. High-throughput sequencing was done using HiSeq 2500 (Illumina, San Diego, CA, USA) as paired-end 100 bp sequencing.

Software tools (TopHat, Toronto, ON, Canada) were used to map RNA-Seq reads. Transcript assembly and detection of differentially expressed genes or isoforms were performed from the alignment file using cufflinks [19]. The quantile normalization method was used for comparison between samples [20]. Functional gene classification was done using Medline databases (http://www.ncbi.nlm.nih.gov/), DAVID (http://david.abcc.ncifcrf.gov/), GenMAPP (http://www.genmapp.org/), and BioCarta (http://www.biocarta.com/) [21]. Pathway analysis was performed on differentially expressed genes [22]. A fold-change of 1.3 and a log2-normalized read count of 4 were the thresholds applied for this study [23].

2.5. Statistical Analysis

All statistical analysis was performed using SPSS 12 for Windows (SPSS Inc., Chicago, IL, USA). A one-way analysis of variance with Tukey's post-hoc test was used to evaluate the differences between each group after performing a test of normality. A *p*-value less than 0.05 was set as the threshold for statistical significance.

3. Results

3.1. Formation of Cell Spheroids with Human Gingiva-Derived Stem Cells

Spheroids were well-established in each microwell on Day 1 (Figure 2). Furthermore, no noticeable changes in the shape of the cell spheroids were observed with the addition of BMP-4 at concentrations of 2, 6, or 10 ng/mL. There were no noticeable changes at the longer culturing times. The spheroid diameters are shown in Figure 3. There was a general decrease in the diameter of the spheroids with longer incubation time.

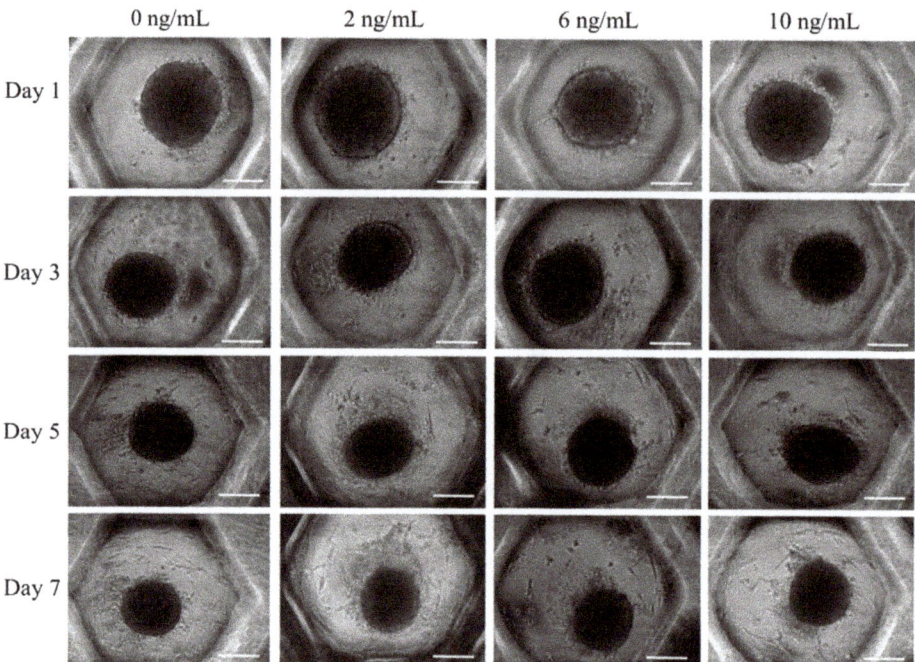

Figure 2. Spheroid morphology on Days 1, 3, 5, and 7. The scale bar indicates 200 μm.

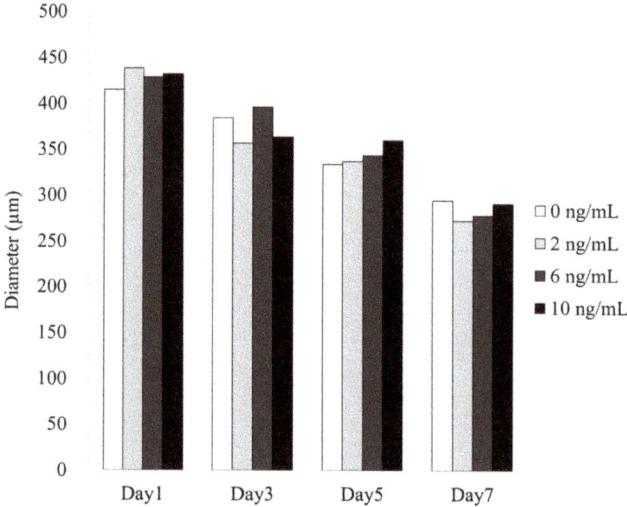

Figure 3. Diameter of the spheroids on Days 1, 3, 5, and 7. The spheroids were treated with BMP-4 at concentrations of 0, 2, 6, or 10 ng/mL.

3.2. Determination of Cellular Viability

Figure 4A shows qualitative results for the viability of cell spheroids at Day 3 using a Live/Dead assay kit (Figure 4A). In all cases, the cells in the spheroids produced intense green fluorescence. Red fluorescence was partly noted around the boundary of the spheroids. No significant differences were noted at Day 7 when compared with results of Day 3 (Figure 4B). Figure 4C shows the quantitative results for cellular viability on Days 1, 3, 5, and 7. No significant differences were observed among the groups on Day 1 ($p > 0.05$). In general, there were no significant differences among the groups with longer incubation times.

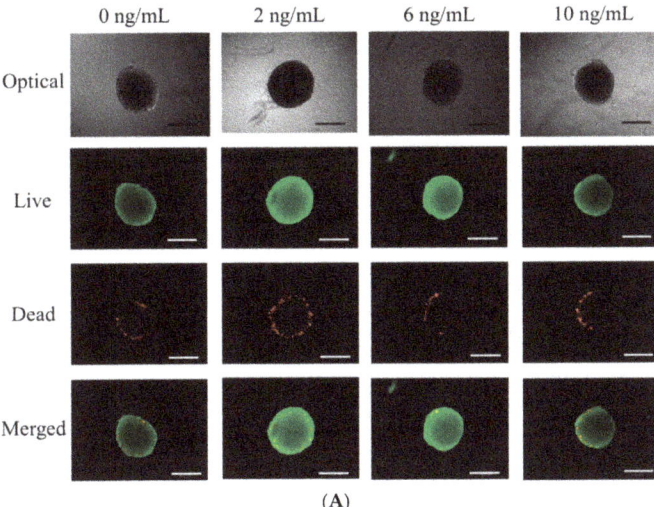

Figure 4. *Cont.*

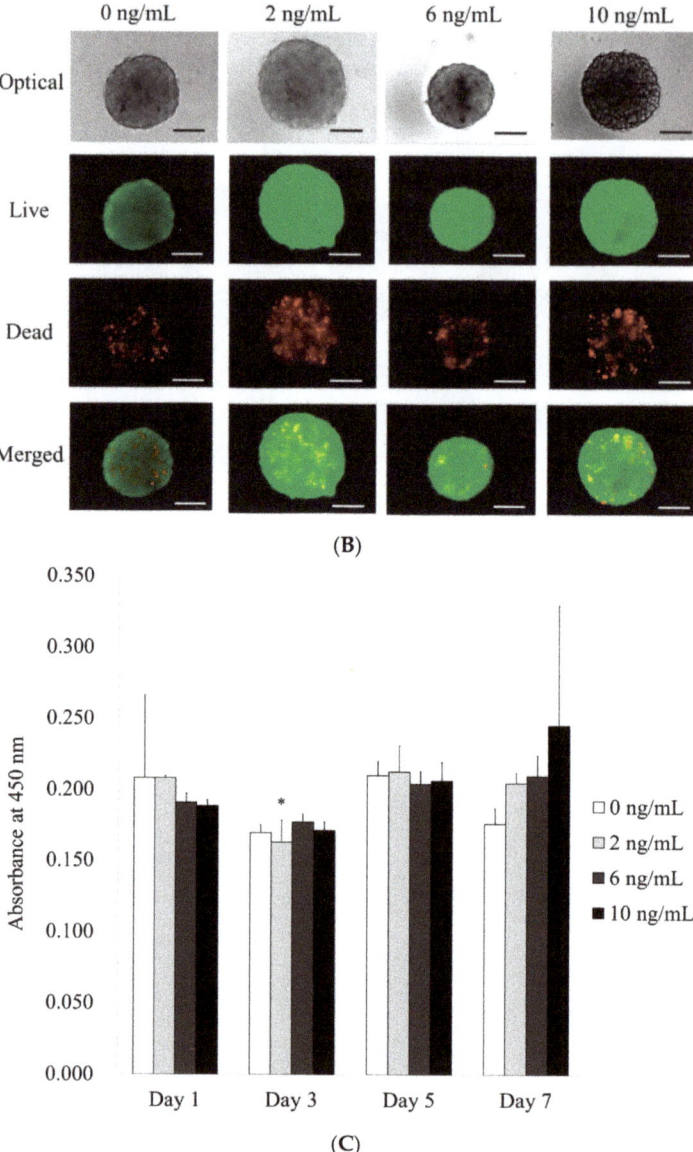

Figure 4. (**A**) Optical, live, dead, and merged images of stem cell spheroids on Day 3. The scale bar indicates 200 μm. (**B**) Results of optical, live, dead, and merged images of stem cell spheroids on Day 7. The scale bar represents 200 μm. (**C**) Cellular viability using CCK-8 assay on Days 1, 3, 5, and 7. * Statistically significant differences were noted when compared with the 2 ng/mL group on Day 1 ($p < 0.05$).

3.3. Evaluation of Alkaline Phosphatase Activity Assay with the Addition of BMP-4

The results of the alkaline phosphatase activity assay at Days 1, 3, 5, and 7 are presented in Figure 5. In general, there were increases in the alkaline phosphatase activity with longer incubation time up to Day 7. Notably, the group treated with 2 ng/mL BMP-4 at Day 3 had a significantly higher activity compared with that of the control group at Day 3 ($p < 0.05$).

3.4. Gene Ontology

A total of 25,737 mRNAs were differentially expressed. Scatter plots of the differentially expressed mRNAs are shown in Figure 6. A Venn diagram of the gene ontology analysis of differentially expressed mRNAs is shown in Figure 7. When compared with the 0 ng/mL control group, 1270 mRNAs were upregulated and 1070 mRNAs were downregulated in the 2 ng/mL group. In the 6 ng/mL group, 1536 mRNAs were upregulated and 1889 mRNAs were downregulated compared to controls. In the 10 ng/mL group, 1525 mRNAs were upregulated and 1533 mRNAs were downregulated compared to controls. A clustering analysis of differentially expressed mRNAs related to osteoblast differentiation is shown in Figure 8. The changes in expression of RUNX2 and CTNNB1 are shown in Figure 9. While the expression of CTNNB1 was increased dose-dependently, the expression of RUNX2 was highest at 6 ng/mL and the expression decreased at the higher dose of 10 ng/mL (Figure 9A,B). The phosphoinositide-3-kinase–protein kinase B/Akt (PI3K/AKT) signaling pathway was involved in the target genes chosen for stem cell differentiation (Figure 10).

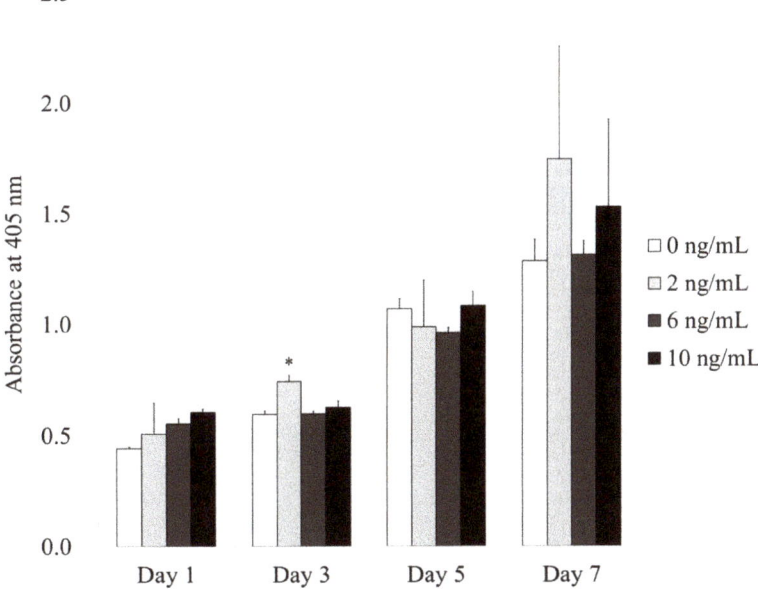

Figure 5. Alkaline phosphatase activity on Days 1, 3, 5, and 7. * Statistically significant differences were noted when compared with the 0 ng/mL group on Day 3 ($p < 0.05$).

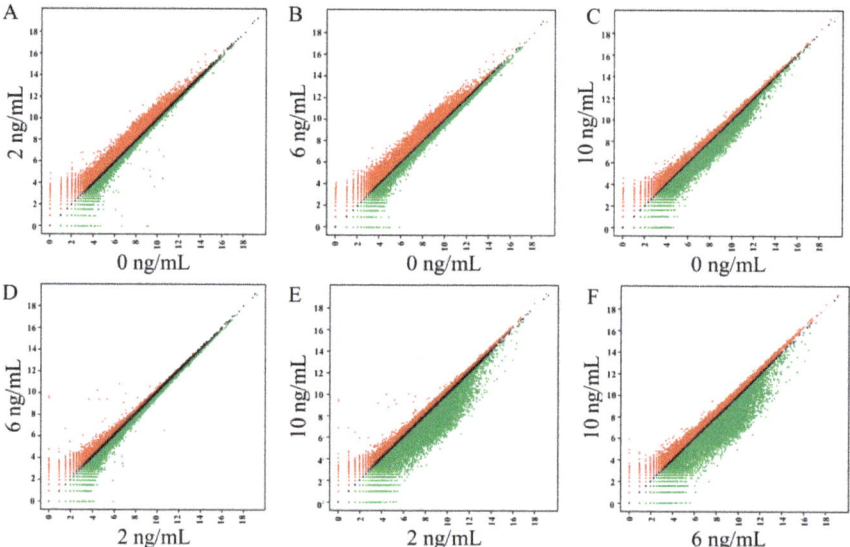

Figure 6. Scatter plots showing the expression of BMP-4 at 0, 2, 6, and 10 ng/mL (x, y-axis: Relative expression level; red indicates that the expression level of the y-value is higher than that of the x-value and green indicates that the expression level of the y-value is lower than that of the x-value). (**A**) 2/0, (**B**) 6/0, (**C**) 10/0, (**D**) 6/2, (**E**) 10/2, and (**F**) 10/6 ng/mL.

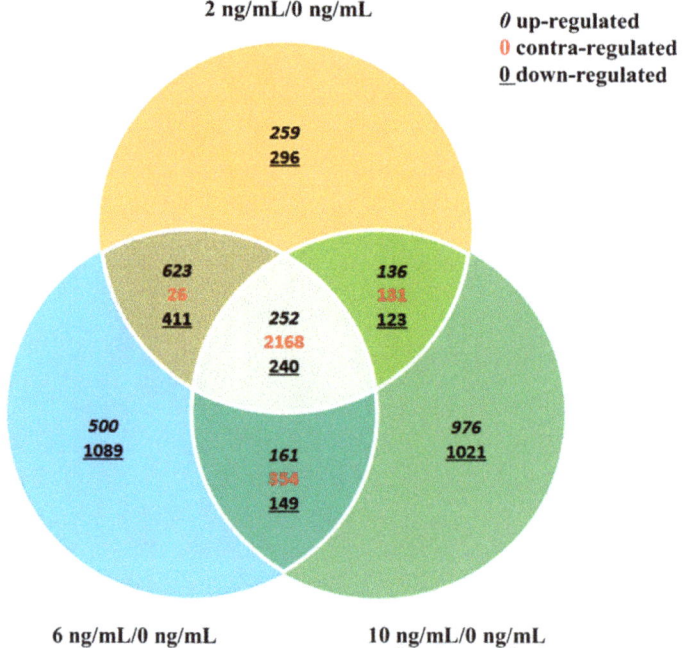

Figure 7. Venn diagram analysis (fold change, 1.3, log2-normalized read counts of 4 were selected).

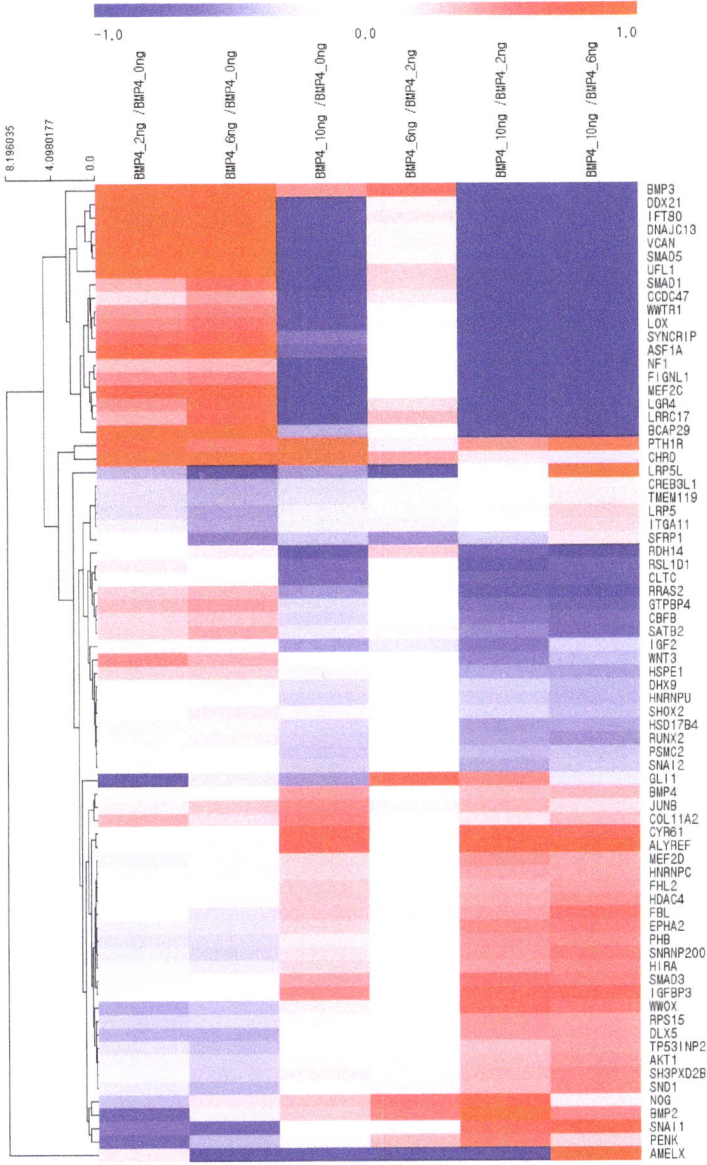

Figure 8. The results of clustering analysis of differentially expressed mRNAs related to osteoblast differentiation (fold change 1.3, log2-normalized read counts of 4 were selected).

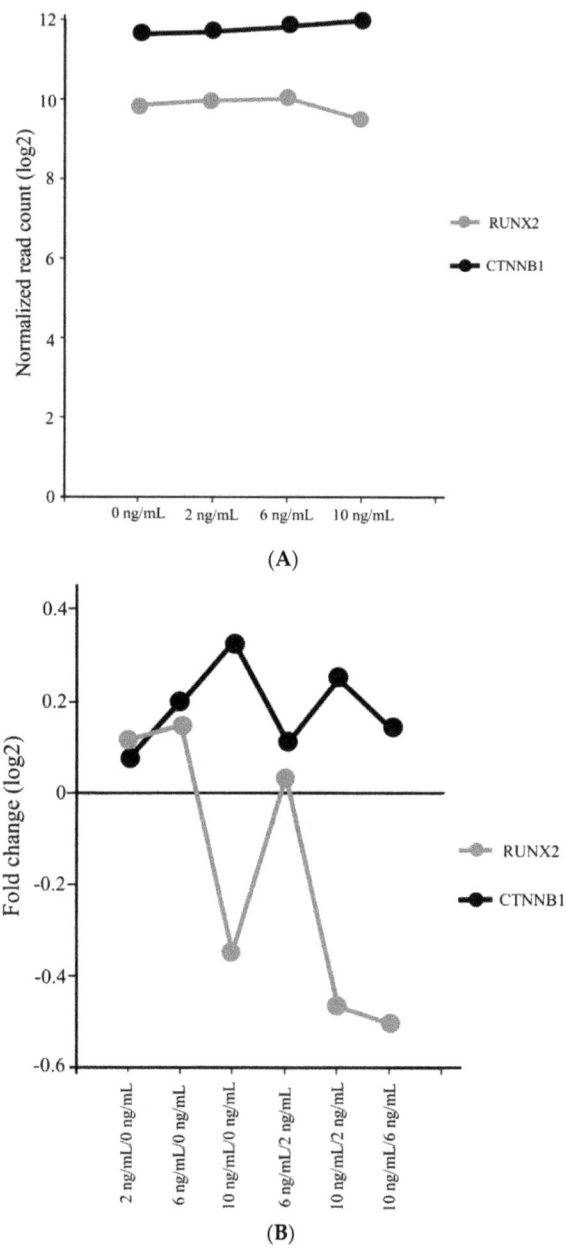

Figure 9. (**A**) Log2-normalized read counts regarding the expression of RUNX2 and CTNNB1. (**B**) Log2 fold change regarding the expression of RUNX2 and CTNNB1.

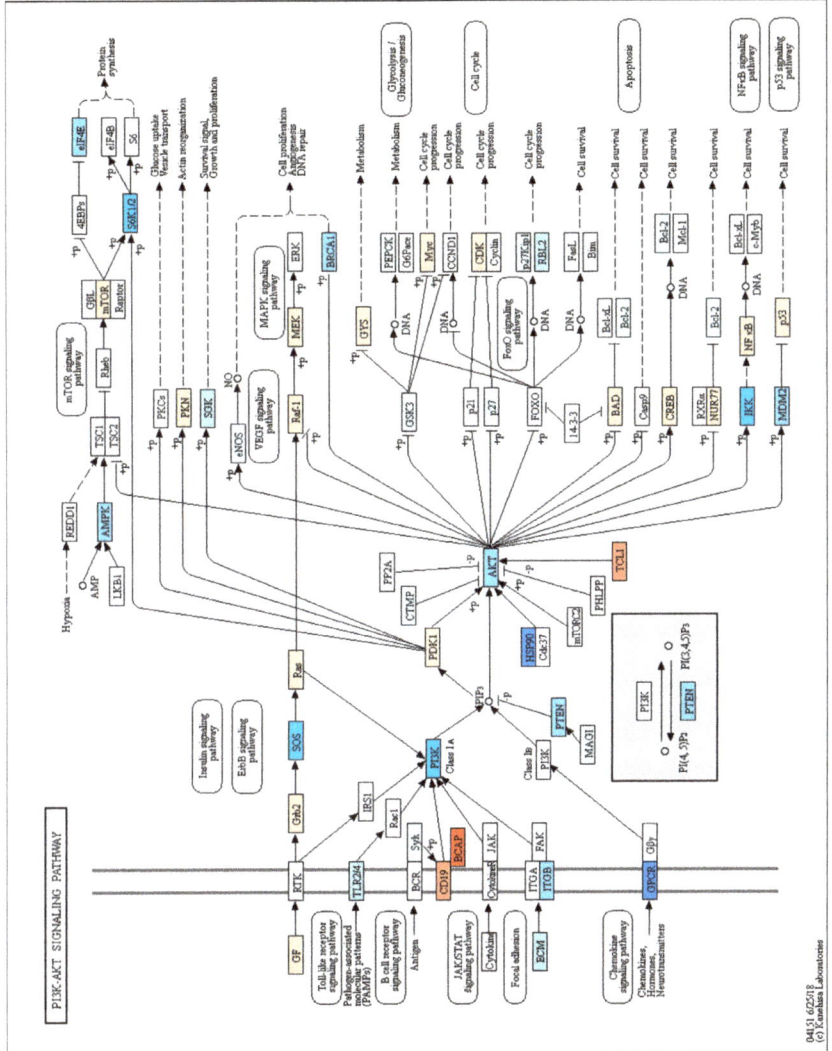

Figure 10. PI3K-AKT signaling pathway.

4. Discussion

In this study, we examined the effects of BMP-4 on stem cell spheroids under predetermined concentrations of 2, 6, and 10 ng/mL and found that the application of BMP-4 increased alkaline phosphatase activity and the expression of RUNX2 and CTNNB1 without affecting cellular viability.

BMP-4 is reported to act as a regulator for osteogenic differentiation and has been shown to induce endochondral and intra-membranous bone formation [12,24]. In a previous report, BMP-4 carried by liposomes seemed to improve the healing process in alveolar bone [25]. Similarly, the expression of BMP-4 appeared to be associated with normal bone homeostasis and the remodeling of grafted and nongrafted maxillary sites [26]. Additionally, BMP-4 induced osteogenic differentiation of mouse skin-derived fibroblasts and dermal papilla cells [24]. Furthermore, a study testing the effects of abnormal BMP-4 expression in the blood of diabetic participants found that low expression of BMP-4 hindered the osteogenic function of bone marrow-derived stem cells [27]. This study also clearly showed that BMP-4 increased osteogenic differentiation of stem cell spheroids composed of gingiva-derived mesenchymal stem cells.

The effects of BMP-4 concentration were tested in previous reports [24,28–32]. Application of 20 ng/mL BMP-4 to primary osteoblastic cells derived from the calvaria resulted in an enhancement in fibronectin synthesis [28]. Treatment with 70 ng/mL of BMP-4 stimulated vascular endothelial growth factor (VEGF) synthesis in osteoblasts [29]. Similarly, the use of 30 ng/mL BMP-4 was associated with an increase in osteoprotegerin synthesis in osteoblast-like MC3T3-E1 cells [30]. At a concentration of 50 ng/mL, BMP-4 induced osteogenic differentiation of mouse skin-derived fibroblasts and dermal papilla cells [24]. Treatment with 500 ng/mL BMP-4 resulted in in vitro osteogenic differentiation of C2C12 cells derived from mouse muscle [31]. Primary human mesenchymal stem cells were treated with 100, 200, or 500 ng/mL BMP-4 and cells were stained with Alizarin red to detect calcium deposition, and the results showed that the 500 ng/mL dose produced the highest value [32]. Moreover, MG63 and Sao2 osteosarcoma cell lines were treated with 25 ng/mL BMP-4 to evaluate the cell cycle distributions, and the results showed that BMP-4 seemed to increase the percent of cells in the G0/G1 phases and decrease the percent of cells in the synthetic and/or G2/M phases [33]. This study showed that the application of 2 or 6 ng/mL BMP-4 could increase the osteogenic differentiation of stem cell spheroids and the expression of related genes. The variety of effects seen across concentrations may be partly due to the differences in cell types, culture conditions, and culture times [34,35].

In a previous report, modification of the roughened anodized titanium implant was done by wet coating with growth factors [36]. In another study, the coating of the titanium implants was obtained by absorption of growth factors after coating the surface with the collagen [17]. The results showed that coating with collagen, chondroitin sulphate, and BMP-4 showed the highest bone-to-implant contact. Enhanced coating can be obtained by applying various methods including chemical bonding, polymer layer, and covering layer [37].

BMP-4 has been proposed to act on various pathways [38–40]. A previous report showed that BMP-4 affected the osteogenic differentiation and mineralization of bone marrow-derived stem cells through Wnt/β-catenin activation [38]. This study suggested the involvement of the PI3K/AKT pathway, and a previous report showed that the mineralization of osteoblasts occurred through the PI3K/AKT pathway [40].

Sequencing was performed to measure genome-wide mRNA expression levels and to investigate the possible mechanisms behind the observed effects of BMP-4. RUNX2 and CTNNB1 (which affect β-catenin expression) are major regulators for osteoblastic lineage [41,42]. RUNX2 is reported to be essential for osteogenic differentiation and is weakly expressed in uncommitted mesenchymal cells but shows up-regulated expression in preosteoblasts [43]. The expression of the osteoblast marker gene RUNX2 was significantly up-regulated in cell spheroids composed of adipose-derived stem cells [44]. β-catenin is reported to be involved in activation of the osteogenic-related signaling pathway [45,46]. β-catenin is also reported to control the differentiation of bone-forming osteoblasts and bone-resorbing osteoclasts [47]. Furthermore, β-catenin is involved in mediating the viability of osteoblasts [48]. In this report, expression levels of both CTNNB1 and RUNX2 were up-regulated with the application of BMP-4. The focusing on RUNX2 and CTNNB1 expression with agonists may produce enhanced functionality. BMP-4 can be suggested as a coating material for the stem cell culture for enhancing for osteogenic differentiation [49]. Moreover, spheroids can be made with stem cells mixed with BMP-4 or impregnated with BMP using fibers [50].

5. Conclusions

This study evaluated the effects of BMP-4 on cellular viability, osteogenic differentiation, and global mRNA expression using stem cell spheroids composed. Together, these results revealed that the application of BMP-4 increased alkaline phosphatase activity and CTNNB1 and RUNX2 expression without affecting cellular viability. Based on this research, the coating with BMP-4 can be applied when stem cells are utilized. BMP-4 can be suggested as a coating material for stem cell cultures. Spheroids impregnated with BMP-4 can be suggested for the bone regeneration field as stem cell therapy.

Author Contributions: Conceptualization, J.-Y.T., Y.-H.P., Y.K. and J.-B.P.; methodology J.-Y.T., Y.-H.P. and J.-B.P.; validation, J.-Y.T., Y.-H.P. and J.-B.P.; formal analysis, J.-Y.T., Y.-H.P. and J.-B.P.; writing—original draft preparation, J.-Y.T., Y.-H.P., Y.K. and J.-B.P.; and writing—review and editing, J.-Y.T., Y.-H.P., Y.K. and J.-B.P. All authors have read and agreed to the published version of the manuscript.

Funding: This study was funded by the National Research Foundation of Korea (NRF) grant funded by the Korea government (MSIT) (No. 2020R1A2C4001624). This research was also funded by Research Fund of Seoul St. Mary's Hospital, The Catholic University of Korea.

Conflicts of Interest: The authors have no competing interests regarding this study.

References

1. Castro-Manrreza, M.E.; Montesinos, J.J. Immunoregulation by mesenchymal stem cells: Biological aspects and clinical applications. *J. Immunol. Res.* **2015**, *2015*, 394917. [CrossRef] [PubMed]
2. Lee, S.-I.; Yeo, S.-I.; Kim, B.-B.; Ko, Y.; Park, J.-B. Formation of size-controllable spheroids using gingiva-derived stem cells and concave microwells: Morphology and viability tests. *Biomed. Rep.* **2016**, *4*, 97–101. [CrossRef]
3. Lee, S.-I.; Ko, Y.; Park, J.-B. Evaluation of the shape, viability, stemness and osteogenic differentiation of cell spheroids formed from human gingiva-derived stem cells and osteoprecursor cells. *Exp. Ther. Med.* **2017**, *13*, 3467–3473. [CrossRef] [PubMed]
4. Watt, F.M.; Driskell, R.R. The therapeutic potential of stem cells. *Philos Trans. R. Soc. Lond. B Biol. Sci.* **2010**, *365*, 155–163. [CrossRef] [PubMed]
5. Montanez-Sauri, S.I.; Beebe, D.J.; Sung, K.E. Microscale screening systems for 3D cellular microenvironments: Platforms, advances, and challenges. *Cell Mol. Life Sci.* **2015**, *72*, 237–249. [CrossRef]
6. Langhans, S.A. Three-Dimensional in Vitro Cell Culture Models in Drug Discovery and Drug Repositioning. *Front. Pharmacol.* **2018**, *9*, 6.
7. Edmondson, R.; Broglie, J.J.; Adcock, A.F.; Yang, L. Three-dimensional cell culture systems and their applications in drug discovery and cell-based biosensors. *Assay Drug Dev. Technol.* **2014**, *12*, 207–218. [CrossRef] [PubMed]
8. Napolitano, A.P.; Dean, D.M.; Man, A.J.; Youssef, J.; Ho, D.N.; Rago, A.P.; Lech, M.P.; Morgan, J.R. Scaffold-free three-dimensional cell culture utilizing micromolded nonadhesive hydrogels. *Biotechniques* **2007**, *43*, 494–500. [CrossRef] [PubMed]
9. Petrenko, Y.; Syková, E.; Kubinová, Š. The therapeutic potential of three-dimensional multipotent mesenchymal stromal cell spheroids. *Stem Cell Res. Ther.* **2017**, *8*, 94. [CrossRef] [PubMed]
10. He, J.; Han, X.; Wang, S.; Zhang, Y.; Dai, X.; Liu, B.; Liu, L.; Zhao, X. Cell sheets of co-cultured BMP-2-modified bone marrow stromal cells and endothelial progenitor cells accelerate bone regeneration in vitro. *Exp. Ther. Med.* **2019**, *18*, 3333–3340. [CrossRef] [PubMed]
11. Bragdon, B.; Moseychuk, O.; Saldanha, S.; King, D.; Julian, J.; Nohe, A. Bone Morphogenetic Proteins: A critical review. *Cell Signal* **2011**, *23*, 609–620. [CrossRef] [PubMed]
12. Rahman, M.S.; Akhtar, N.; Jamil, H.M.; Banik, R.S.; Asaduzzaman, S.M. TGF-β/BMP signaling and other molecular events: Regulation of osteoblastogenesis and bone formation. *Bone Res.* **2015**, *3*, 15005. [CrossRef] [PubMed]
13. Modica, S.; Wolfrum, C. The dual role of BMP4 in adipogenesis and metabolism. *Adipocyte* **2017**, *6*, 141–146. [CrossRef] [PubMed]
14. Li, Q.; Wijesekera, O.; Salas, S.J.; Wang, J.Y.; Zhu, M.; Aprhys, C.; Chaichana, K.L.; Chesler, D.A.; Zhang, H.; Smith, C.L.; et al. Mesenchymal stem cells from human fat engineered to secrete BMP4 are nononcogenic, suppress brain cancer, and prolong survival. *Clin. Cancer Res.* **2014**, *20*, 2375–2387. [CrossRef]
15. Kang, Q.; Sun, M.H.; Cheng, H.; Peng, Y.; Montag, A.G.; Deyrup, A.T.; Jiang, W.; Luu, H.H.; Luo, J.; Szatkowski, J.P.; et al. Characterization of the distinct orthotopic bone-forming activity of 14 BMPs using recombinant adenovirus-mediated gene delivery. *Gene Ther.* **2004**, *11*, 1312–1320. [CrossRef]
16. Gluhak-Heinrich, J.; Guo, D.; Yang, W.; Harris, M.A.; Lichtler, A.; Kream, B.; Zhang, J.; Feng, J.Q.; Smith, L.C.; Dechow, P.; et al. New roles and mechanism of action of BMP4 in postnatal tooth cytodifferentiation. *Bone* **2010**, *46*, 1533–1545. [CrossRef]

17. Stadlinger, B.; Pilling, E.; Mai, R.; Bierbaum, S.; Berhardt, R.; Scharnweber, D.; Eckelt, U. Effect of biological implant surface coatings on bone formation, applying collagen, proteoglycans, glycosaminoglycans and growth factors. *J. Mater. Sci. Mater. Med.* **2008**, *19*, 1043–1049. [CrossRef]
18. Son, J.; Tae, J.Y.; Min, S.K.; Ko, Y.; Park, J.B. Fibroblast growth factor-4 maintains cellular viability while enhancing osteogenic differentiation of stem cell spheroids in part by regulating RUNX2 and BGLAP expression. *Exp. Ther. Med.* **2020**, *20*, 2013–2020. [CrossRef]
19. Trapnell, C.; Pachter, L.; Salzberg, S.L. TopHat: Discovering splice junctions with RNA-Seq. *Bioinformatics* **2009**, *25*, 1105–1111. [CrossRef]
20. Gentleman, R.C.; Carey, V.J.; Bates, D.M.; Bolstad, B.; Dettling, M.; Dudoit, S.; Ellis, B.; Gautier, L.; Ge, Y.; Gentry, J.; et al. Bioconductor: Open software development for computational biology and bioinformatics. *Genome Biol.* **2004**, *5*, 80. [CrossRef]
21. Huang, D.W.; Sherman, B.T.; Tan, Q.; Collins, J.R.; Alvord, W.G.; Roayaei, J.; Stephens, R.; Baseler, M.W.; Lane, H.C.; Lempicki, R.A. The DAVID Gene Functional Classification Tool: A novel biological module-centric algorithm to functionally analyze large gene lists. *Genome Biol.* **2007**, *8*, 183. [CrossRef] [PubMed]
22. Kanehisa, M.; Furumichi, M.; Tanabe, M.; Sato, Y.; Morishima, K. KEGG: New perspectives on genomes, pathways, diseases and drugs. *Nucleic Acids Res.* **2017**, *45*, 353–361. [CrossRef] [PubMed]
23. Lee, H.; Min, S.K.; Song, Y.; Park, Y.H.; Park, J.B. Bone morphogenetic protein-7 upregulates genes associated with osteoblast differentiation, including collagen I, Sp7 and IBSP in gingiva-derived stem cells. *Exp. Ther. Med.* **2019**, *18*, 2867–2876. [CrossRef] [PubMed]
24. Myllylä, R.M.; Haapasaari, K.M.; Lehenkari, P.; Tuukkanen, J. Bone morphogenetic proteins 4 and 2/7 induce osteogenic differentiation of mouse skin derived fibroblast and dermal papilla cells. *Cell Tissue Res.* **2014**, *355*, 463–470. [CrossRef]
25. Ferreira, C.L.; Abreu, F.A.; Silva, G.A.; Silveira, F.F.; Barreto, L.B.; Paulino Tde, P.; Miziara, M.N.; Alves, J.B. TGF-β1 and BMP-4 carried by liposomes enhance the healing process in alveolar bone. *Arch. Oral Biol.* **2013**, *58*, 646–656. [CrossRef] [PubMed]
26. Torrecillas-Martínez, L.; Galindo-Moreno, P.; Ávila-Ortiz, G.; Ortega-Oller, I.; Monje, A.; Hernández-Cortés, P.; Aguilar, D.; O'Valle, F. Significance of the immunohistochemical expression of bone morphogenetic protein-4 in bone maturation after maxillary sinus grafting in humans. *Clin. Implant Dent. Relat. Res.* **2016**, *18*, 717–724. [CrossRef]
27. Liang, C.; Sun, R.; Xu, Y.; Geng, W.; Li, J. Effect of the abnormal expression of BMP-4 in the blood of diabetic patients on the osteogenic differentiation potential of alveolar BMSCs and the rescue effect of metformin: A bioinformatics-based study. *Biomed. Res. Int.* **2020**, *2020*, 7626215. [CrossRef]
28. Tang, C.H.; Yang, R.S.; Liou, H.C.; Fu, W.M. Enhancement of fibronectin synthesis and fibrillogenesis by BMP-4 in cultured rat osteoblast. *J. Bone Miner Res.* **2003**, *18*, 502–511. [CrossRef]
29. Kondo, A.; Otsuka, T.; Kuroyanagi, G.; Yamamoto, N.; Matsushima-Nishiwaki, R.; Mizutani, J.; Kozawa, O.; Tokuda, H. Resveratrol inhibits BMP-4-stimulated VEGF synthesis in osteoblasts: Suppression of S6 kinase. *Int. J. Mol. Med.* **2014**, *33*, 1013–1018. [CrossRef]
30. Fujita, K.; Otsuka, T.; Yamamoto, N.; Kainuma, S.; Ohguchi, R.; Kawabata, T.; Sakai, G.; Kuroyanagi, G.; Matsushima-Nishiwaki, R.; Kozawa, O.; et al. (−)-Epigallocatechin gallate but not chlorogenic acid upregulates osteoprotegerin synthesis through regulation of bone morphogenetic protein-4 in osteoblasts. *Exp. Ther. Med.* **2017**, *14*, 417–423. [CrossRef]
31. Lee, S.H.; Hwang, J.W.; Han, Y.; Lee, K.Y. Synergistic stimulating effect of 2-hydroxymelatonin and BMP-4 on osteogenic differentiation in vitro. *Biochem. Biophys. Res. Commun.* **2020**, *527*, 941–946. [CrossRef] [PubMed]
32. Lavery, K.; Swain, P.; Falb, D.; Alaoui-Ismaili, M.H. BMP-2/4 and BMP-6/7 differentially utilize cell surface receptors to induce osteoblastic differentiation of human bone marrow-derived mesenchymal stem cells. *J. Biol. Chem.* **2008**, *283*, 20948–20958. [CrossRef]
33. Chang, S.F.; Chang, T.K.; Peng, H.H.; Yeh, Y.T.; Lee, D.Y.; Yeh, C.R.; Zhou, J.; Cheng, C.K.; Chang, C.A.; Chiu, J.J. BMP-4 induction of arrest and differentiation of osteoblast-like cells via p21 CIP1 and p27 KIP1 regulation. *Mol. Endocrinol.* **2009**, *23*, 1827–1838. [CrossRef] [PubMed]
34. van der Sanden, B.; Dhobb, M.; Berger, F.; Wion, D. Optimizing stem cell culture. *J. Cell Biochem.* **2010**, *111*, 801–807. [CrossRef]

35. Kang, S.H.; Park, J.B.; Kim, I.; Lee, W.; Kim, H. Assessment of stem cell viability in the initial healing period in rabbits with a cranial bone defect according to the type and form of scaffold. *J. Periodontal Implant Sci.* **2019**, *49*, 258–267. [CrossRef]
36. Bates, C.; Marino, V.; Fazzalari, N.L.; Bartold, P.M. Soft tissue attachment to titanium implants coated with growth factors. *Clin. Implant Dent. Relat. Res.* **2013**, *15*, 53–63. [CrossRef]
37. Wang, J.; Guo, J.; Liu, J.; Wei, L.; Wu, G. BMP-functionalised coatings to promote osteogenesis for orthopaedic implants. *Int. J. Mol. Sci.* **2014**, *15*, 10150–10168. [CrossRef]
38. Ruan, Y.; Kato, H.; Taguchi, Y.; Yamauchi, N.; Umeda, M. Irradiation by high-intensity red light-emitting diode enhances human bone marrow mesenchymal stem cells osteogenic differentiation and mineralization through Wnt/β-catenin signaling pathway. *Lasers Med. Sci.* **2020**, *25*, 1–11. [CrossRef]
39. Wang, Y.; He, Y.; Cao, Z.; Fang, Y.; Du, M.; Liu, Z. Regulatory effects of bone morphogenetic protein-4 on tumour necrosis factor-α-suppressed Runx2 and osteoprotegerin expression in cementoblasts. *Cell Prolif.* **2017**, *50*, e12344. [CrossRef]
40. Ayala-Peña, V.B.; Scolaro, L.A.; Santillán, G.E. ATP and UTP stimulate bone morphogenetic protein-2,-4 and -5 gene expression and mineralization by rat primary osteoblasts involving PI3K/AKT pathway. *Exp. Cell Res.* **2013**, *319*, 2028–2036. [CrossRef] [PubMed]
41. Vega, O.A.; Lucero, C.M.J.; Araya, H.F.; Jerez, S.; Tapia, J.C.; Antonelli, M.; Salazar-Onfray, F.; Las Heras, F.; Thaler, R.; Riester, S.M.; et al. Wnt/β-Catenin Signaling Activates Expression of the Bone-Related Transcription Factor RUNX2 in Select Human Osteosarcoma Cell Types. *J. Cell Biochem.* **2017**, *118*, 3662–3674. [CrossRef] [PubMed]
42. Tae, J.Y.; Lee, H.; Lee, H.; Ko, Y.; Park, J.B. Osteogenic potential of cell spheroids composed of varying ratios of gingiva-derived and bone marrow stem cells using concave microwells. *Exp. Ther. Med.* **2018**, *16*, 2287–2294. [CrossRef] [PubMed]
43. Hopkins, A.; Mirzayans, F.; Berry, F. Foxc1 Expression in Early Osteogenic Differentiation Is Regulated by BMP4-SMAD Activity. *J. Cell Biochem.* **2016**, *117*, 1707–1717. [CrossRef] [PubMed]
44. Rumiński, S.; Kalaszczyńska, I.; Długosz, A.; Lewandowska-Szumieł, M. Osteogenic differentiation of human adipose-derived stem cells in 3D conditions—Comparison of spheroids and polystyrene scaffolds. *Eur. Cell Mater.* **2019**, *37*, 382–401. [CrossRef]
45. Zhang, J.; He, X.; Chen, X.; Wu, Y.; Dong, L.; Cheng, K.; Lin, J.; Wang, H.; Weng, W. Enhancing osteogenic differentiation of BMSCs on high magnetoelectric response films. *Mater. Sci. Eng. C Mater. Biol. Appl.* **2020**, *113*, 110970. [CrossRef]
46. Kim, B.B.; Kim, M.; Park, Y.H.; Ko, Y.; Park, J.B. Short-term application of dexamethasone on stem cells derived from human gingiva reduces the expression of RUNX2 and β-catenin. *J. Int. Med. Res.* **2017**, *45*, 993–1006. [CrossRef]
47. Kramer, I.; Halleux, C.; Keller, H.; Pegurri, M.; Gooi, J.H.; Weber, P.B.; Feng, J.Q.; Bonewald, L.F.; Kneissel, M. Osteocyte Wnt/beta-catenin signaling is required for normal bone homeostasis. *Mol. Cell Biol.* **2010**, *30*, 3071–3085. [CrossRef]
48. Chu, Y.; Gao, Y.; Yang, Y.; Liu, Y.; Guo, N.; Wang, L.; Huang, W.; Wu, L.; Sun, D.; Gu, W. β-catenin mediates fluoride-induced aberrant osteoblasts activity and osteogenesis. *Environ. Pollut.* **2020**, *265*, 114734. [CrossRef]
49. Liu, D.; Pavathuparambil Abdul Manaph, N.; Al-Hawwas, M.; Bobrovskaya, L.; Xiong, L.L.; Zhou, X.F. Coating Materials for Neural Stem/Progenitor Cell Culture and Differentiation. *Stem Cells Dev.* **2020**, *29*, 463–474. [CrossRef]
50. Ahmad, T.; Byun, H.; Lee, J.; Madhurakat Perikamana, S.K.; Shin, Y.M.; Kim, E.M.; Shin, H. Stem cell spheroids incorporating fibers coated with adenosine and polydopamine as a modular building blocks for bone tissue engineering. *Biomaterials* **2020**, *230*, 119652. [CrossRef]

Publisher's Note: MDPI stays neutral with regard to jurisdictional claims in published maps and institutional affiliations.

© 2020 by the authors. Licensee MDPI, Basel, Switzerland. This article is an open access article distributed under the terms and conditions of the Creative Commons Attribution (CC BY) license (http://creativecommons.org/licenses/by/4.0/).

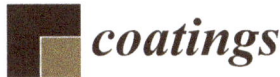

Article

The Impact of Curcumin on Bone Osteogenic Promotion of MC3T3 Cells under High Glucose Conditions and Enhanced Bone Formation in Diabetic Mice

Jia He [1], Xiaofeng Yang [1], Fan Liu [1], Duo Li [1], Bowen Zheng [1], Adil Othman Abdullah [2,3,*] and Yi Liu [1,*]

1. Department of Orthodontics, School of Stomatology, China Medical University, Liaoning Provincial Key Laboratory of Oral Diseases, Shenyang 110002, China; jiahe@cmu.edu.cn (J.H.); xfyang90@cmu.edu.cn (X.Y.); fanliu@cmu.edu.cn (F.L.); duoli@cmu.edu.cn (D.L.); bwzheng@cmu.edu.cn (B.Z.)
2. School of Stomatology, China Medical University, Liaoning Provincial Key Laboratory of Oral Diseases, Shenyang 110002, China
3. Prosthodontics Department, Erbil Polytechnic University, Kurdistan Region, Erbil 44001, Iraq
* Correspondence: adil.abdullah@epu.edu.iq (A.O.A.); liuyi@cmu.edu.cn (Y.L.); Tel.: +964-7504604246 (A.O.A.); +86-24-3197-3999 (Y.L.)

Received: 6 February 2020; Accepted: 7 March 2020; Published: 10 March 2020

Abstract: Diabetic osteoporosis (DOP) is characterized by impaired bone microstructure and reduced bone density resulting from high glucose levels. Curcumin (CURC) is extensively applied in the treatment of inflammation-associated diseases. However, the effect of curcumin on bone metabolism in diabetic osteoporosis is unclear. Therefore, this study investigated the optimal concentration of curcumin on enhancing osteogenesis in diabetic osteoporosis. Osteoblasts were treated with a high or low concentration of curcumin under a series of concentrations of high-glucose conditions. Type 2 diabetic mice were intervened with curcumin. Cell proliferation, apoptosis, and osteogenesis-related gene expressions were evaluated by CCK-8, flow cytometry, and real-time quantitative reverse transcription polymerase chain reaction (RT-qPCR). Bone formation was evaluated by histological staining. The findings revealed that curcumin suppressed apoptosis and enhanced proliferation and osteogenesis-related gene expressions of osteoblasts under high glucose concentrations ($p < 0.05$). The histological sections displayed reduced bone destruction and increased the growth rate of trabecular bone and the bone density of diabetic mice treated with curcumin, compared to diabetic mice. These results showed that curcumin could reverse the harmful effects of diabetic osteoporosis in a dose-dependent manner, and 10 µmol/L was regarded as the optimal concentration, which supports the potential use of curcumin for bone regeneration under high glucose concentrations.

Keywords: curcumin; high glucose; osteogenesis; bone formation; diabetic osteoporosis

1. Introduction

Diabetes mellitus is characterized by hyperglycemia caused by decreased insulin sensitivity or insulin deficiency [1], which has been regarded as a significant risk factor that threatens human health. Based on the statistical reports from the International Diabetes Federation (IDF), approximately 451 million diabetic patients suffered from diabetic complications in 2017 [2]. More seriously, the number is predicted to significantly increase to 590 million by 2035. Among various diabetic complications, diabetic osteoporosis (DOP) results in low bone mass, impaired bone microstructure, and reduced bone mineral density (BMD) [3,4]. Research has demonstrated a more than 60% higher incidence of bone fracture in diabetic patients than that of unaffected patients [5–7]. More importantly, the delayed union of bone fracture after surgery in clinic severely affects patients' physical function and even mental health.

The traditional method for the therapy of type 2 diabetes mellitus is to inject insulin to reduce blood glucose levels, but therapy has hardly promoted bone formation [8]. Polypeptides, hormones, and genes are also used locally as bioactive molecules to enhance bone formation. However, the instable status, risk of an immunological inflammatory response, and the high cost of these molecules need to be carefully studied [9–11].

Recent investigations have focused on natural components that have no related side effects and promote osteoimmunomodulation at low cost [12]. Curcumin (CURC), derived from the plant *Curcuma longa*, is a bioactive component of turmeric with the ability to modulate the immune system [13]. Although curcumin has poor water solubility and low bioavailability and stability, some studies have confirmed that drug carriers such as proteins, polymeric particles, and polylactic-glycolic acid copolymer (PLGA) microspheres can effectively solve this problem and give full play to its antioxidant, anti-inflammatory, and anti-hyperglycemic properties [14–18]. Natural or chemically modified curcumin could upregulate insulin sensitivity and reduce glucose and glycosylated hemoglobin levels, which has great potential as an alternative therapeutic option for diabetes mellitus and its complications [19,20]. More importantly, it is reported that curcumin could suppress osteoclast activities by inhibiting the expression of transcription factor AP-1 [21]. Moreover, curcumin, in combination with insulin, inhibits alveolar bone loss of experimental periodontitis in diabetic rats [22].

Although several studies have reported the effect of curcumin on diabetic bone formation [23,24], there is a lack of scientific information on the concentration of curcumin and its toxicity. The concentration of glucose in vitro has also not been systematically investigated. Thus, it is important to confirm the optimal concentration of curcumin and its effect on osteogenesis under a series of high glucose concentrations.

Therefore, our study investigated the optimal concentration of curcumin, its toxicity, and osteogenic effect on osteogenesis of osteoblasts under a series of glucose concentrations in vitro. The bone density and growth rate of type 2 diabetic mice in the presence of curcumin were evaluated by histological sections.

2. Materials and Methods

2.1. In Vitro Analysis

2.1.1. Cell Culture

Mouse osteoblast precursor MC3T3 cells were obtained from the American Type Culture Collection (ATCC, Manassas, VA, USA) and cultured in α-MEM (Hyclone Laboratories, Inc., Logan, UT, USA) containing 10% fetal bovine serum (FBS) (Gemini Bio-Products, West Sacramento, CA, USA) and 1% streptomycin (Hyclone). Osteogenic differentiation medium contained 10% FBS, 1% streptomycin, 1% dexamethasone (Sigma-Aldrich, St. Louis, MO, USA), 50 μg/mL L-ascorbic acid (Sigma-Aldrich), and 10 mmol/L β-sodium glycerophosphate (Sigma-Aldrich.) and was used for osteogenic differentiation tests. The cells were cultured at 37 °C with 5% CO_2. The culture medium was replaced every 2 days until the cells reached 80%–100% confluence. Experiment groups were divided based on the concentrations of curcumin and glucose, which are listed in Table 1.

Table 1. Experiment groups and abbreviations.

Experiment Groups	Glucose	Curcumin	Abbreviation
Control	5.5 mmol/L	0 μmol/L	C
Medium glucose	11 mmol/L	0 μmol/L	Mg
High glucose	16.5 mmol/L	0 μmol/L	Hg
Medium glucose/Low curcumin	11 mmol/L	5 μmol/L	Mg-Lc
Medium glucose/High curcumin	11 mmol/L	10 μmol/L	Mg-Hc
High glucose/Low curcumin	16.5 mmol/L	5 μmol/L	Hg-Lc
High glucose/High curcumin	16.5 mmol/L	10 μmol/L	Hg-Hc

2.1.2. Cell Proliferation

Cell viability was determined by a Cell Counting Kit-8 (Beyotime, Shanghai, China). The MC3T3-E1 cells were seeded at 2×10^3 cells per well in 96-well culture plates for 24, 48, and 72 h. At the above time points, the cells were washed twice with PBS solution, and 250 μL fresh culture medium with 25 μL CCK-8 reagent was sequentially added to each sample. After incubation for 2 h at 37 °C, 100 μL medium was transferred to a 96-well plate and measured at 450 nm by using a micro-plate reader (Infinite M200, Tecan, Männedorf, Switzerland).

2.1.3. Cell Apoptosis

Annexin V-fluoroisothiocyanate (FITC)/propidium iodide (PI) double staining (Dojindo, Japan) was used to determine cell apoptosis. Cells were seeded at 1×10^6 cells per well in 6-well plates and cultured in growth media for 24 h. Subsequently, the medium was replaced with fresh growth medium containing different concentrations of glucose and curcumin as described above. After 48 h, cells were stained with PI and Annexin V-FITC in a dark room for 15 min, according to manufacturer instructions, and analyzed by flow cytometry (Cytomics FC 500 MCL, Beckman Coulter, Brea, CA, USA).

2.1.4. Osteogenesis-Related Gene Expression of MC3T3 Cells

Quantitative real-time reverse transcription polymerase chain reaction (qRT-PCR) was performed to determine the osteogenic gene expression of MC3T3. Cells were seeded at 1.5×10^5 cells/well under different concentrations of glucose and curcumin. The total RNA from all groups was first extracted using the RNAiso plus kit (Takara Bio, Japan), determined with a NanoDrop ND-1000 spectrophotometer (NanoDrop Technologies, Wilmington, NC, USA), and was reversed to cDNA by the Reverse Transcription Kit (Takara Bio, Tokyo, Japan). The RT-qPCR was performed using a SYBR green kit and specific primers (Dalian Bao Biological Takara Corporation, Dalian, China) via the StepOnePlus™ Real-Time PCR system (Thermo Fisher Scientific, Shanghai, China). Primers are as follows: Runx2, forward 5'-CATTTGCACTGGGTCACACGTA-3', reverse 5'-GAATCTGGCCATGTTTGTGCTC-3' (159 bp); *Opn* forward 5'- TACGACCATGAGATTGGCAGTGA-3', reverse 5'- TATAGGATCTGGGTGCAGGCTGTAA-3' (127 bp); Col-1 forward 5'-GTGGCGGTTATGACTTCAGC-3', reverse 5'-TCACGAACAACGTTAGCATC-3' (154 bp); GAPDH forward 5'-TTCGACAGTCAGCCGCATCTT-3', reverse 5'- ATCCGTTGACTCCGACCTTCA-3' (145 bp). The PCR reactions were activated at 95 °C for 30 s, followed by an amplification target sequence of 40 cycles at 95 °C for 5 s, 60 °C for 34 s, and 95 °C for 15 s. The relative expression levels of the genes were calculated by the 2−ΔΔCT method.

2.2. In Vivo Analysis

2.2.1. Experimental Animals and Grouping

The protocol was approved by the Ethical Committee and the Laboratory Animal Center of China medical university, Shenyang, Liaoning, China. Eighteen 10-week-old specific pathogen-free (SPF) male mice from the Jackson Laboratory (Bar Harbor, ME, USA) were maintained at a constant temperature (22–25 °C) in a 12 h light/dark cycle and fed with a standard laboratory diet and water.

Six non-diabetic BLKS/jdb/m male mice were selected as the control group (db/m, $n = 6$, weight: 18.4–10.7 g). Twelve spontaneous diabetic BLKS/jdb/db male mice were randomly separated into the diabetic group (db/db, $n = 6$, weight: 35.9–40.9 g) and the curcumin-treated diabetic group (db/db + C, $n = 6$, weight: 35.7–40.3 g). Each group was kept in the same cage. The curcumin-treated group was intragastrically given a dose of 200 mg/kg/d curcumin for 10 weeks, and the control group and diabetic group were given equivalent volumes of solution (normal saline + 0.1% DMSO) for 10 weeks. Curcumin was dissolved in DMSO, then diluted with normal saline to make the content of DMSO 0.1% and administered daily by gavage. All groups were sacrificed at 20 weeks, and mandibles (3 mm × 3 mm) were harvested and fixed in 4% paraformaldehyde solution for 7 days at 4 °C in the dark. The Block sections were sequentially dehydrated in ascending serial concentrations of ethanol, cleared with xylene twice, and embedded in poly(methyl methacrylate). Serial sections with a thickness of 70–80 μm were cut parallel to the coronal plane and prepared for fluorescence microscopy and histological staining. All analyses of in vivo experiments were made by an experienced pathologist (blind to the treatments of the mice) in order to characterize any changes.

2.2.2. Polyfluorochrome Sequential Labeling of Bone

Bone formation was assessed by sequential labeling with Calcein and tetracycline (Sigma-Aldrich), which were deposited at the active site of mineralization. The fluorochromes were administered by intraperitoneal injection in the following sequence: calcein (20 mg/kg) was added to 2% $NaHCO_3$ buffer and given to three 19-week-old mice randomly selected from each group ($n = 9$). Four days later, the same mice were injected with tetracycline (30 mg/kg) in 0.9% normal saline. The sections were observed by fluorescence microscopy.

2.2.3. Histological Analysis

The osteogenesis effect of curcumin treatment in diabetic mice was evaluated by Masson's Trichrome staining (Beyotime). The sections were preserved in well-prepared Weigert's hematoxylin solution for 10 min. After rinsing with running tap water and acetified water, the slides were firstly stained by Masson Fuchsin Acid Complex for 5 min, then immersed in 2% glacial acetic acid solution, 1% phosphomolybdic acid, 2% aniline blue, and 0.2% acetic acid in sequence. Finally, sections were fixed into neutral gum for microscopy observation.

2.3. Statistical Analysis

GraphPad Prism 5.0 software (San Diego, CA, USA) was utilized to perform statistical analysis. The quantitative data were depicted as mean ± standard deviation ($n = 3$). One-way ANOVA and multi-way ANOVA were used to calculate the statistical significance among glucose-treated groups and curcumin-treated groups, respectively. Statistically significant differences between each two groups at each time point were evaluated using the t-test. A p value of less than 0.05 was considered statistically significant.

3. Results and Discussion

Previous studies have demonstrated high glucose inhibits proliferation and differentiation of osteoblasts [25]. Curcumin promotes osteogenic differentiation of osteoblasts [26]. The concentration of curcumin at 15 μmol/L showed a stronger osteogenic effect than that at 10 μmol/L, whereas it was not statistically significant, and the concentration of curcumin at 25 μmol/L showed obvious cytotoxicity [27,28]. Therefore, we grouped within the concentration range of 10μmol/l in our study. In addition, curcumin can induce cancerous cell apoptosis in specific doses and times through different pathways. However, it does not have a significant effect on normal cells in the same doses/times, which suggests that sensitivity of cells to curcumin varies under different conditions [28]. Therefore, the protective effect of curcumin on high glucose-induced apoptosis and the optimal concentration of curcumin in promoting osteogenesis in diabetic osteoporosis under different glucose concentrations are still unclear. Our findings proved that curcumin effectively alleviates high glucose-induced negative effects on osteoblasts, its optimal concentration, and osteogenic impact on osteogenesis of osteoblasts under a series of glucose concentrations.

3.1. Effect of Curcumin on the Viability of MC3T3 Cells in High-Glucose Conditions

The proliferation of MC3T3 treated by curcumin under different concentrations of glucose was investigated by using a CCK-8 kit at 24, 48, and 72 h. No differences could be found among each group at 24 h. Cell viability in the control group increased most up to 48 h, and was significantly higher than that in the other groups ($p < 0.05$). The high-glucose group had the lowest cell viability, indicating that a higher concentration of glucose severely affected cell viability. When curcumin was introduced, cell viabilities in different glucose groups significantly increased ($p < 0.05$), whereas there were no differences between low and high concentrations of curcumin treatment. At 72 h, the cell viability in the curcumin-treated groups was significantly higher than that in the glucose groups ($p < 0.05$; Figure 1). Three concentrations of glucose were selected in present study. At 16.5 mmol/L glucose, there was a negative influence on cell viability. No differences were found on the effect of concentrations of curcumin among curcumin-treated groups.

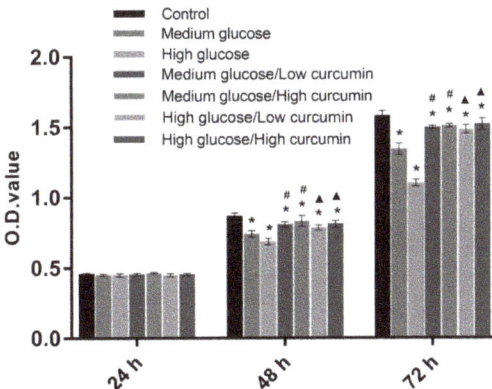

Figure 1. Effects of curcumin on viability of MC3T3 cells in high-glucose conditions. Cell viability was measured using the CCK8 assay after culturing for 24, 48, and 72 h, separately. The bar chart shows the mean optical density (OD) values ($n = 3$). *$p < 0.05$ vs the control group; #$p < 0.05$ vs the medium glucose group; ▲$p < 0.05$ vs the high-glucose group.

3.2. Effect of Curcumin on Apoptosis of MC3T3 Cells in High-Glucose Conditions

Flow cytometry showed that curcumin treatment had an effect on glucose-induced apoptosis in MC3T3 cells (Figure 2A). The first-quadrant cells were necrotic and consisted of late apoptotic cells, which could be simultaneously stained with Annexin V-FITC and PI. The second-quadrant cells were PI-negative. In the third quadrant, normal living cells were not stained with Annexin V-FITC or PI. The fourth-quadrant cells were only stained with Annexin V-FITC, indicating early apoptotic cells. The early apoptosis rates of the control and glucose groups were 9.03% ± 0.67%, 14.70% ± 0.26%, and 18.70% ± 0.61%, and the curcumin-treated groups were 13.30% ± 0.10%, 12.00% ± 0.85%, 16.80% ± 0.20%, and 13.77% ± 0.21%. Glucose significantly increased the rate of apoptosis ($p < 0.05$), whereas treatment with both low and high doses of curcumin significantly decreased the apoptosis rate for cells under different concentrations of glucose ($p < 0.05$). In the high glucose group, the apoptosis rate in the high concentration of the curcumin group was significantly lower than that in the low concentration of the curcumin group ($p < 0.05$; Figure 2B), whereas there were no differences in the medium glucose group. It can be concluded that treatment with curcumin significantly protected cells from hyperglycemia-triggered apoptosis of MC3T3 cells under high-glucose conditions. This was shown in a dose-dependent manner under a high concentration of glucose, but not under a low concentration of glucose, under which a low concentration of curcumin can achieve an optimal protective effect on cells. This expands on previous observations that curcumin mitigates hyperglycemia-related clinical symptoms [29,30].

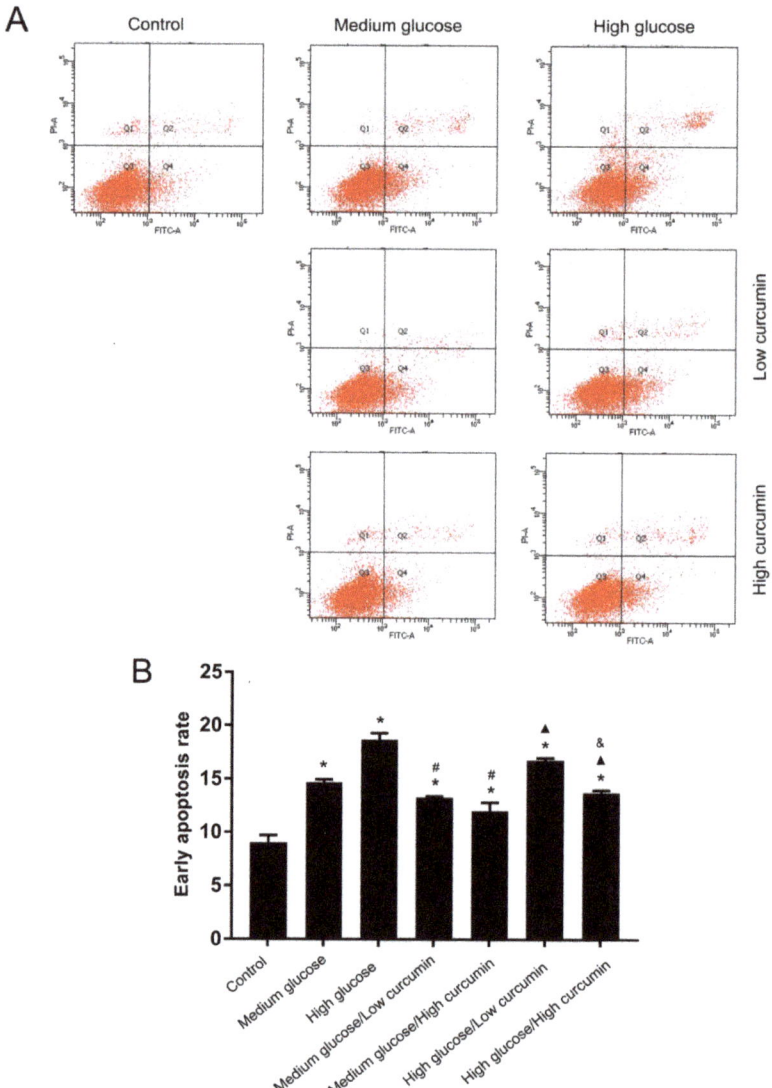

Figure 2. Effects of curcumin on apoptosis of MC3T3 cells in high-glucose conditions. Cell apoptosis was assessed by staining the cells with Annexin V-FITC/PI double staining kit and subsequent analysis by flow cytometry. (**A**) Detection of the early apoptosis rate of MC3T3 cells using flow cytometry. (**B**) The bar chart shows the mean of early apoptosis rate ($n = 3$). *$p < 0.05$ vs the control group; #$p < 0.05$ vs the medium glucose group; ▲$p < 0.05$ vs the high glucose group; and &$p < 0.05$ vs the high glucose/low curcumin group.

3.3. Effect of Curcumin on Osteogenic Differentiation of MC3T3 Cells in Glucose Conditions

The expressions of osteogenesis-related genes Runx2, Opn, and Col-1 in MC3T3 cells related to different concentrations of glucose and curcumin were evaluated using real-time quantitative PCR (RT-qPCR). Runx2 is crucial for osteoblastogenesis, regulates the differentiation, maturation, and bone formation of osteoblasts, and activates the expression of other osteogenic genes, such as Col-1 during early stages and Opn during late stages [31,32]. Col-1 is an important organic component of the bone matrix and the most crucial extracellular protein in bone, which initially provides a structural framework for inorganic deposition [33]. Opn is a phosphorylated glycoprotein secreted by osteoblasts and can promote biomineralization and bone remodeling [18]. In addition, the specific binding of Opn to Col-1 may naturally localize Opn, influencing the adhesion, differentiation, and function of osteoblasts [34]. In the present study, the expressions of Runx2, Opn, and Col-1 genes were significantly downregulated in the high glucose-treated group and were significantly lower than those of the control and medium glucose-treated groups ($p < 0.05$), indicating that a higher concentration of glucose severely affected expression of osteogenesis-related genes. When curcumin was introduced, the expressions of Runx2, Opn, and Col-1 genes were significantly upregulated at different concentrations of glucose ($p < 0.05$). The expressions of Runx2 and Col-1 genes in the high curcumin-treated group were significantly higher than those in the low curcumin-treated group ($p < 0.05$), whereas there was no significant difference in the expression of Opn between the low and high curcumin-treated groups (Figure 3). The results demonstrated that the osteogenic effect of curcumin was dose-dependent in the early stage of osteogenesis, but not in the late stage. It is possible that curcumin might predominantly upregulate the expression of Runx2, which in turn enhanced Col-1 expression in precursor osteoblasts, whereas Opn has a unique regulation mechanism, which is different from the combination of Col-1 and Runx2. It is interesting to further investigate the mechanism of curcumin upregulating Runx2, Opn, and Col-1 expressions in osteoblasts and the relationship between the expression of each gene. The current results indicated that curcumin could induce differentiation of MC3T3 cells from pre-osteoblasts to osteoblasts in different concentrations of glucose in a dose-dependent manner. Curcumin could serve as an effective method to recover glucose-suppressed osteogenic differentiation in precursor osteoblasts. In addition, 10 μmol/L curcumin was found to be an effective concentration that could promote osteogenic differentiation of MC3T3 under different concentrations of glucose.

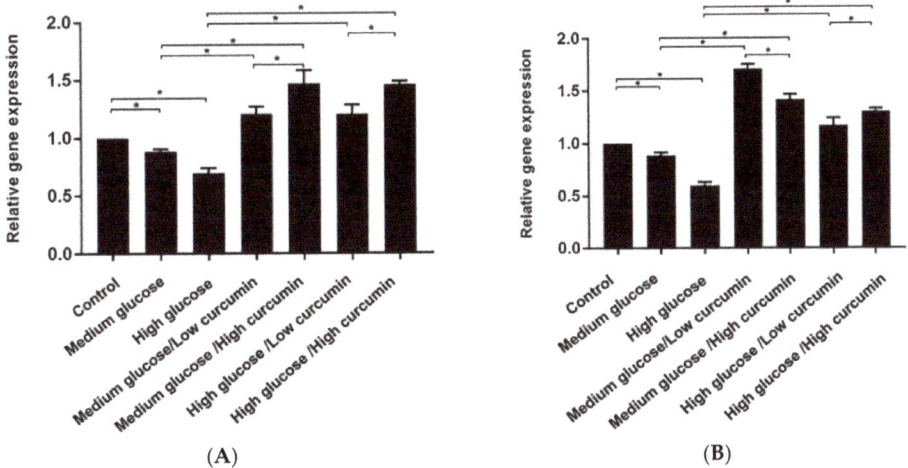

Figure 3. Cont.

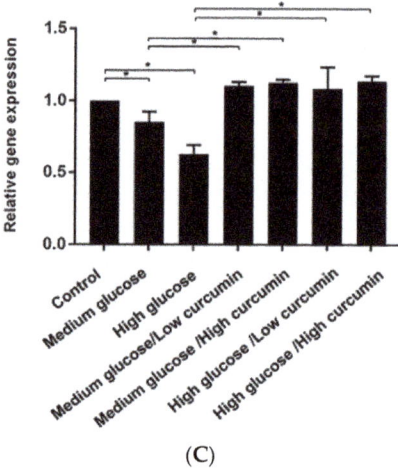

(C)

Figure 3. Effects of curcumin on osteogenic differentiation of MC3T3 cells in glucose conditions. Expressions of (**A**) Runx2, (**B**) Opn, and (**C**) Col-1 were measured by reverse transcription quantitative polymerase chain reaction (RT-qPCR; $n = 3$). The results are shown as a relative expression level of the target gene using glyceraldehyde-3-phosphate-dehydrogenase (GAPDH) as the inner reference gene, and analyzed by 2-$\Delta\Delta$Ct. Data are shown as mean ± SD. *$p < 0.05$.

3.4. Curcumin Treatment Improved Alveolar Bone Formation in Diabetic Mice

Diabetes mellitus (DM) is a significant risk factor for osteoporosis. The proliferation and differentiation of osteoblasts in the alveolar bone of diabetic patients remains highly relevant in the daily work of dentists, as they can impact treatment for many oral diseases such as dental implants and oral surgery. Hyperglycemia is often displayed in diabetic patients and has a negative effect on alveolar bone reconstruction [35].

Previous studies have suggested a positive effect of curcumin on bone formation in diabetes and diabetes-related periodontitis [22]. However, few studies have investigated the effectiveness of natural curcumin on alveolar bone formation in diabetic osteoporosis, and there is also a lack of investigations into cortical bone and cancellous bone.

The present study evaluated cortical and cancellous bones by fluorescent double-labeling and Masson staining, respectively. The results revealed that significant differences in alveolar bone loss were observed in curcumin-treated groups when compared with diabetic mice. A general observation from fluorescence images (Figure 4A) was that curcumin treatment significantly enhanced alveolar cortical bone continuity and thickness when compared to diabetic mice, which was similar to that of non-diabetic mice. A general observation from Masson staining (Figure 4C) was that curcumin treatment extremely enhanced alveolar cancellous bone density and mineralization in diabetic mice, which is similar to that of non-diabetic mice. Curcumin treatment significantly enhanced the trabecular bone formation rate compared to diabetic mice (1.60 ± 0.11 um/d (diabetic) vs. 0.55 ± 0.05 um/d (curcumin), $p < 0.05$), and there was no significant difference observed when compared to the non-diabetic group (1.18 ± 0.11 um/d (non-diabetic)) (Figure 4B). These results show that curcumin treatment could improve alveolar bone structure in diabetes, and this is in agreement with the results of osteogenesis of MC3T3-E1 cells in response to curcumin treatment in vitro.

Diabetic hyperglycemia can trigger excessive production of ROS and increase oxidative stress, which leads to damaged macromolecular substances (nucleic acids and lipids), induction of cell apoptosis, and inhibition of osteogenic differentiation [36]. Bone protective effects of curcumin on diabetic mice may be explained by reducing the production of ROS induced by high glucose, enhancing antioxidant defense, and even further regulating the osteoimmunological RANK/RANKL/OPG pathway, which inhibits the expression of RANKL and promotes the expression of OPG in osteoblasts, results in an increase in bone formation and a decrease in bone resorption, thus offsetting the negative effects caused by high-glucose conditions. However, the specific mechanism remains to be confirmed by further research.

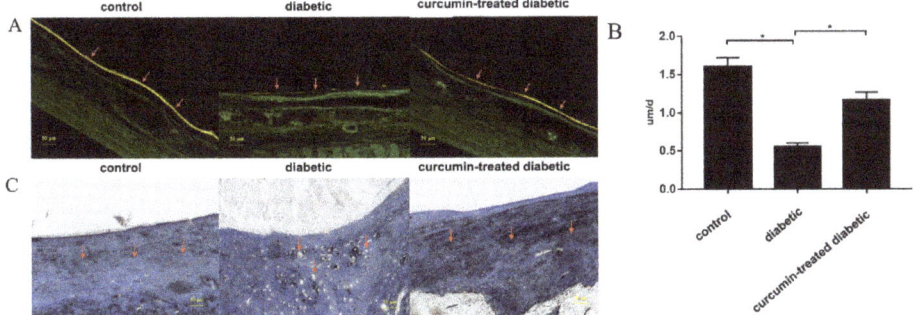

Figure 4. Evaluation of the osteogenic effect of curcumin on bone formation in vivo. (**A**) Fluorescent microscopy images of alveolar bone in non-diabetic (control), diabetic, and curcumin-treated groups, respectively. Alveolar cortical bone continuity and thickness improved in the db/db + C group compared with that in the db/db group, which was similar to that of the db/m group. (**B**) The bar chart shows the rate of trabecular formation. *$p < 0.05$. (**C**) Masson staining images of alveolar bone in non-diabetic (control), diabetic, and curcumin-treated groups, respectively. Alveolar cancellous bone density and mineralization improved in the db/db + C group compared with that in the db/db group, which was similar to that of the db/m group.

4. Conclusions

The results demonstrated that curcumin could protect cells from high glucose-mediated cytotoxicity, promote osteogenic differentiation of mouse precursor MC3T3 cells in a dose-dependent manner, and significantly improve alveolar bone formation in type 2 diabetic mice. These findings provide new insights into the pathogenesis of diabetes-related osteoporosis and indicate that curcumin may be valuable for prevention and inhibition of diabetes-related osteoporosis, providing a theoretical basis for the clinical treatment of alveolar bone disease in diabetic patients.

Author Contributions: All authors had equal contribution to this paper and research. Conceptualization, J.H. and X.Y.; Data curation, J.H. and A.O.A.; Formal analysis, D.L. and B.Z.; Investigation, J.H. and X.Y.; Supervision, Y.L.; Writing—original draft, J.H.; Writing—review and editing, F.L., A.O.A., and Y.L. All authors have read and agreed to the published version of the manuscript.

Funding: This research was funded by the Liaoning Province Natural Science with grant No. (20180550420), and Liaoning province key research and development guidance plan project with grant No. (2019 JH8/10300015).

Acknowledgments: The authors would like to express their thanks to teachers and students in the Experimental Centre of School and Hospital of Stomatology, China Medical University, for their continuous help and support.

Conflicts of Interest: The authors declare no conflicts of interest.

References

1. Zhang, N.; Du, S.M.; Ma, G.S. Current lifestyle factors that increase risk of T2DM in China. *Eur. J. Clin. Nutr.* **2017**, *71*, 832–838. [CrossRef] [PubMed]
2. Guariguata, L.; Whiting, D.R.; Hambleton, I.; Beagley, J.; Linnenkamp, U.; Shaw, J.E. Global estimates of diabetes prevalence for 2013 and projections for 2035. *Diabetes Res. Clin. Pract.* **2014**, *103*, 137–149. [CrossRef] [PubMed]
3. Wu, T.; Qiao, S.; Shi, C.; Wang, S.; Ji, G. Metabolomics window into diabetic complications. *J. Diabetes Investig.* **2018**, *9*, 244–255. [CrossRef] [PubMed]

4. De Amorim, L.M.N.; Vaz, S.R.; Cesário, G.; Coelho, A.S.G.; Botelho, P. Effect of green tea extract on bone mass and body composition in individuals with diabetes. *J. Funct. Foods* **2018**, *40*, 589–594. [CrossRef]
5. Wang, T.; Cai, L.; Wang, Y.; Wang, Q.; Lu, D.; Chen, H.; Ying, X. The protective effects of silibinin in the treatment of streptozotocin-induced diabetic osteoporosis in rats. *Biomed. Pharmacother.* **2017**, *89*, 681–688. [CrossRef]
6. Hamann, C.; Kirschner, S.; Günther, K.P.; Hofbauer, L.C. Bone, sweet bone-osteoporotic fractures in diabetes mellitus. *Nat. Rev. Endocrinol.* **2012**, *8*, 297–305. [CrossRef]
7. Schwartz, A.V. Efficacy of osteoporosis therapies in diabetic patients. *Calcif. Tissue Int.* **2017**, *100*, 165–173. [CrossRef]
8. Onishi, Y.; Yamada, K.; Zacho, J.; Ekelund, J.; Iwamoto, Y. Insulin degludec/insulin aspart versus biphasic insulin aspart 30 twice daily in Japanese subjects with type 2 diabetes: A randomized controlled trial. *J. Diabetes Investig.* **2017**, *8*, 210–217. [CrossRef]
9. Wang, W.; Liu, H.; Xiao, S.; Liu, S.; Li, X.; Yu, P. Effects of insulin plus glucagon-like peptide-1 receptor agonists (GLP-1RAs) in treating type 1 diabetes mellitus: A systematic review and meta-analysis. *Diabetes Ther.* **2017**, *8*, 727–738. [CrossRef]
10. Eibich, P.; Green, A.; Hattersley, A.T.; Jennison, C.; Lonergan, M.; Pearson, E.R.; Gray, A.M. Costs and treatment pathways for type 2 diabetes in the UK: A mastermind cohort study. *Diabetes Ther.* **2017**, *8*, 1031–1045. [CrossRef]
11. Xie, A.; Li, R.; Tao, J.; Jiang, T.; Yan, H.; Zhang, H.; Yang, Y.; Yang, L.; Yechoor, V.; Chan, L.; et al. Anti-TCRβ mAb in combination with Neurogenin3 gene therapy reverses established overt type 1 diabetes in female NOD mice. *Endocrinology* **2017**, *158*, 3140–3151. [CrossRef] [PubMed]
12. Elburki, M.S.; Moore, D.D.; Terezakis, N.G.; Zhang, Y.; Lee, H.M.; Johnson, F.; Golub, L.M. A novel chemically modified curcumin reduces inflammation-mediated connective tissue breakdown in a rat model of diabetes: Periodontal and systemic effects. *J. Periodontal. Res.* **2017**, *52*, 186–200. [CrossRef] [PubMed]
13. Alessandra, G.M.; Daniela, F.P.; Jossiele, W.L.; Tamiris, R.S.; Pedro, H.D.; Matheus, H.J.; Vania, L.L.; Daniela, B.R.L. Hyperlipidemia-induced lipotoxicity and immune activation in rats are prevented by curcumin and rutin. *Int. Immunopharmacol.* **2020**, *81*, 106217. [CrossRef]
14. Busari, Z.A.; Dauda, K.A.; Morenikeji, O.A.; Afolayan, F.; Oyeyemi, O.T.; Meena, J.; Sahu, D.; Panda, A.K. Antiplasmodial activity and toxicological assessment of curcumin PLGA-encapsulated nanoparticles. *Front. Pharmacol.* **2017**, *8*, 622. [CrossRef] [PubMed]
15. Ziwei, M.; Na, W.; Haibing, H.; Xing, T. Pharmaceutical strategies of improving oral systemic bioavailability of curcumin for clinical application. *J. Control. Release* **2019**, *31*, 359–380. [CrossRef]
16. Vincenzo, D.L.; Sante, D.G.; Francesco, M.; Paola, F.; Roberto, C.; Erminia, M.; Angela, A.; Massimo, C.; Lucia, C. Eudragit S100 entrapped liposome for curcumin delivery: Anti-oxidative effect in Caco-2 cells. *Coatings* **2020**, *10*, 114. [CrossRef]
17. Anita, B.; Inese, M.; Simons, S.; Modra, M.; Martins, K. Curcumin effect on copper transport in HepG2 cells. *Medicina* **2018**, *54*, 14. [CrossRef]
18. Abbassy, M.A.; Watari, I.; Soma, K. The effect of diabetes mellitus on rat mandibular bone formation and microarchitecture. *Eur. J. Oral. Sci.* **2010**, *118*, 364–369. [CrossRef]
19. Naijil, G.; Anju, T.R.; Jayanarayanan, S.; Paulose, C.S. Curcumin pretreatment mediates antidiabetogenesis via functional regulation of adrenergic receptor subtypes in the pancreas of multiple low-dose streptozotocin-induced diabetic rats. *Nutr. Res.* **2015**, *35*, 823–833. [CrossRef]
20. Elburki, M.S.; Rossa, C.J.; Guimaraes-stabili, M.R.; Lee, H.M.; Curylofo, F.A.; Johnson, F.; Golub, L.M. A chemically modified curcumin (CMC 2.24) inhibits nuclear factor κB activation and inflammatory bone loss in murine models of LPS-induced experimental periodontitis and diabetes-associated natural periodontitis. *Inflammation* **2017**, *40*, 1436–1449. [CrossRef]
21. Wu, T.J.; Lin, C.Y.; Tsai, C.H.; Huang, Y.L.; Tang, C.H. Glucose suppresses IL-1β-induced MMP-1 expression through the FAK, MEK, ERK, and AP-1 signaling pathways. *Environ. Toxicol.* **2018**, *33*, 1061–1068. [CrossRef] [PubMed]
22. Pimentel, S.P.; Casati, M.Z.; Ribeiro, F.V.; Corrêa, M.G.; Franck, F.C.; Benatti, B.B.; Cirano, F.R. Impact of natural curcumin on the progression of experimental periodontitis in diabetic rats. *J. Periodontal Res.* **2019**. [CrossRef] [PubMed]

23. Yu, L.; Zhanzhao, Z. Sustained curcumin release from PLGA microspheres improves bone formation under diabetic conditions by inhibiting the reactive oxygen species production. *Drug Des. Dev. Ther.* **2018**, *12*, 1453–1466. [CrossRef]
24. Cirano, F.R.; Pimentel, S.P.; Casati, M.Z.; Corrêa, M.G.; Pino, D.S.; Messora, M.R.; Silva, P.H.F.; Ribeiro, F.V. Effect of curcumin on bone tissue in the diabetic rat: Repair of peri-implant and critical-sized defects. *Int. J. Oral. Maxillofac. Surg.* **2018**, *47*, 1495–1503. [CrossRef] [PubMed]
25. Yang, L.; Liu, J.; Shan, Q.; Geng, G.; Shao, P. High glucose inhibits proliferation and differentiation of osteoblast in alveolar bone by inducing pyroptosis. *Biochem. Biophys. Res. Commun.* **2020**, *522*, 471–478. [CrossRef] [PubMed]
26. Son, H.E.; Kim, E.J.; Jang, W.G. Curcumin induces osteoblast differentiation through mild-endoplasmic reticulum stress-mediated such as BMP2 on osteoblast cells. *Life Sci.* **2018**, *193*, 34–39. [CrossRef]
27. Yang, H.; Gu, Q.; Huang, C.; Shi, Q.; Cai, Y. Curcumin increases rat mesenchymal stem cell osteoblast differentiation but inhibits adipocyte differentiation. *Pharmacogn. Mag.* **2012**, *8*, 202–208. [CrossRef]
28. Chang, R.; Sun, L.; Webster, T.J. Short communication: Selective cytotoxicity of curcumin on osteosarcoma cells compared to healthy osteoblasts. *Int. J. Nanomed.* **2014**, *9*, 461–465. [CrossRef]
29. Moran, J.M.; Roncero-Martin, R.; Rodriguez-Velasco, F.J.; Calderon-Garcia, J.F.; Rey-Sanchez, P.; Vera, V.; Canal-Macias, M.L.; Pedrera-Zamorano, J.D. Effects of curcumin on the proliferation and mineralization of human osteoblast-like cells: Implications of nitric oxide. *Int. J. Mol. Sci.* **2012**, *13*, 16104–16118. [CrossRef]
30. Notoya, M.; Nishimura, H.; Woo, J.T.; Nagai, K.; Ishihara, Y.; Hagiwara, H. Curcumin inhibits the proliferation and mineralization of cultured osteoblasts. *Eur. J. Pharmacol.* **2006**, *534*, 55–62. [CrossRef]
31. Corrêa, M.G.; Pires, P.R.; Ribeiro, F.V.; Pimentel, S.Z.; Casarin, R.C.; Cirano, F.R.; Tenenbaum, H.T.; Casati, M.Z. Systemic treatment with resveratrol and/or curcumin reduces the progression of experimental periodontitis in rats. *J. Periodontal Res.* **2017**, *52*, 201–220. [CrossRef] [PubMed]
32. Boșca, A.B.; Ilea, A.; Soriţău, O.; Tatomir, C.; Mikláśová, N.; Pârvu, A.E.; Mihu, C.M.; Melincovici, C.S.; Fischer-Fodor, E. Modulatory effect of curcumin analogs on the activation of metalloproteinases in human periodontal stem cells. *Eur. J. Oral. Sci.* **2019**, *127*, 304–312. [CrossRef] [PubMed]
33. Dong, M.; Jiao, G.; Liu, H.; Wu, W.; Li, S.; Wang, Q.; Xu, D.; Li, X.; Liu, H.; Chen, Y. Biological silicon stimulates collagen type 1 and osteocalcin synthesis in human osteoblast-like cells through the BMP-2/Smad/RUNX2 signaling pathway. *Biol. Trace Elem. Res.* **2016**, *173*, 306–315. [CrossRef] [PubMed]
34. Foster, B.L.; Ao, M.; Salmon, C.R.; Chavez, M.B.; Kolli, T.N.; Tran, A.B.; Chu, E.Y.; Kantovitz, K.R.; Yadav, M.; Narisawa, S. Osteopontin regulates dentin and alveolar bone development and mineralization. *Bone* **2018**, *107*, 196–207. [CrossRef] [PubMed]
35. Colombo, J.S.; Balani, D.; Sloan, A.J.; Crean, S.J.; Okazaki, J.; Waddington, R.J. Delayed osteoblast differentiation and altered inflammatory response around implants placed in incisor sockets of type 2 diabetic rats. *Clin. Oral. Implants Res.* **2011**, *22*, 578–586. [CrossRef]
36. Fakhruddin, S.; Alanazi, W.; Jackson, K.E. Diabetes-induced reactive oxygen species: Mechanism of their generation and role in renal injury. *J. Diabetes Res.* **2017**, *2017*, 1–30. [CrossRef]

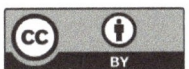

© 2020 by the authors. Licensee MDPI, Basel, Switzerland. This article is an open access article distributed under the terms and conditions of the Creative Commons Attribution (CC BY) license (http://creativecommons.org/licenses/by/4.0/).

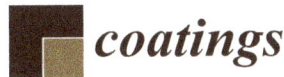

Article

Cytotoxicity and Mineralization Potential of Four Calcium Silicate-Based Cements on Human Gingiva-Derived Stem Cells

Donghee Lee [1,†], Jun-Beom Park [2,†], Dani Song [3], Hye-Min Kim [3] and Sin-Young Kim [3,*]

1. College of Medicine, The Catholic University of Korea, Seoul 06591, Korea; dong524@naver.com
2. Department of Periodontics, College of Medicine, The Catholic University of Korea, Seoul 06591, Korea; jbassoon@catholic.ac.kr
3. Department of Conservative Dentistry, Seoul St. Mary's Dental Hospital, College of Medicine, The Catholic University of Korea, Seoul 06591, Korea; eksl0104@gmail.com (D.S.); hmtoto@naver.com (H.-M.K.)
* Correspondence: jeui99@catholic.ac.kr; Tel.: +82-2-2258-1787
† These authors contributed equally to this study.

Received: 10 February 2020; Accepted: 16 March 2020; Published: 18 March 2020

Abstract: The aim of this study was to evaluate the cytotoxicity and mineralization potential of four calcium silicate-based cements on human gingiva-derived stem cells (GDSCs). The materials evaluated in the present study were ProRoot MTA (Dentsply Tulsa Dental Specialties), Biodentine (Septodont), Endocem Zr (Maruchi), and RetroMTA (BioMTA). Experimental disks of 6 mm in diameter and 3 mm in height were produced and placed in a 100% humidified atmosphere for 48 h to set. We evaluated the cytotoxic effects of the cements using methyl-thiazoldiphenyl-tetrazolium (MTT) and live/dead staining assays. We used a scratch wound healing assay to evaluate cell migratory ability. Mineralization potential was determined with an Alizarin red S (ARS) staining assay. In the MTT assay, no significant differences were found among the ProRoot MTA, Biodentine, and control groups during the test period ($p > 0.05$). The Endocem Zr and RetroMTA groups showed relatively lower cell viability than the control group at day 7 ($p < 0.05$). In the wound healing assay, no significant differences were found among the ProRoot MTA, Biodentine, Endocem Zr, and control groups during the test period ($p > 0.05$). The RetroMTA group had slower cell migration compared to the control group at days 3 and 4 ($p < 0.05$). In the ARS assay, the ProRoot MTA, Biodentine, and RetroMTA groups exhibited a significant increase in the formation of mineralized nodules compared to the Endocem Zr and control groups on day 21 ($p < 0.05$). In conclusion, the four calcium silicate-based cements evaluated in the present study exhibited good biological properties on GDSCs. ProRoot MTA, Biodentine, and RetroMTA showed higher mineralization potential than the Endocem Zr and control groups.

Keywords: cell survival; cell migration assay; calcium silicate-based cements; calcium nodule formation

1. Introduction

External root resorption (ERR) happens when the periodontal ligament of the cementum is either destructed or removed [1]. Damage to the cementum uncovers the root surface to osteoclasts that can resorb dentin. With additional stimulation provoked by sulcular bacteria in the neighboring area, root resorption constantly progresses [2]. ERR of a permanent tooth is generally unfavorable because it may cause irreversible damage and ultimately loss of the tooth. However, in its early stages, ERR can be stabilized by repairing the cementum with calcium silicate-based cement [3].

Calcium silicate-based cements are hydraulic materials consisting of tricalcium silicate, dicalcium silicate, and tricalcium aluminate [4,5]. The first tricalcium silicate-based cement was mineral trioxide aggregate (MTA), which is a derivative of Portland cement. The physical, chemical, and biological properties of MTA have been studied for decades, and it produces favorable results when applied to direct pulp capping, regenerative endodontic procedure, apical retrograde filling, and repair of ERR or perforations [6]. Tricalcium silicate enhances proliferation and differentiation of dental pulp cells [7–9]. However, ProRoot MTA (Dentsply Tulsa Dental Specialties, Tulsa, OK, USA) contains heavy metal components such as bismuth oxide [5]. It also has a long setting time and handling difficulty, and can discolor the tooth and gingiva [10,11]. Novel calcium silicate-based cements have been produced overcome these shortcomings.

Biodentine (Septodont, Saint-Maur-des-Fossés, France) is composed mostly of tricalcium silicate, zirconium oxide, and calcium carbonate powder, which are mixed with a supplied solution that includes calcium chloride [12,13]. The reduced setting time compared to MTA is achieved by diminishing the particle size and adding calcium chloride to expedite the reactions [13–15]. The substitution of bismuth oxide with zirconium oxide may also play a role in reduced setting time, because this component has been reported to expedite the primary hydration reaction [13]. Previous studies of this material's effects on dental pulp stem cells demonstrated its biocompatible ability, odontoblast differentiation ability, and mineralization potential [12,16]. Endocem Zr (Maruchi, Wonju, Korea) and RetroMTA (BioMTA, Seoul, Korea) were developed to cause less tooth discoloration compared to ProRoot MTA [17]. These materials have a reduced setting time compared to ProRoot MTA and are easy to handle [18,19]. Bismuth oxide is replaced by zirconium oxide as a substitute radiopacifier [17]. RetroMTA is composed of fine hydrophilic particles that do not originate from Portland cement [19].

To the best of our knowledge, no study has evaluated the biocompatibility and calcium nodule formation ability of various calcium silicate-based cements on human gingiva-derived stem cells (GDSCs). Therefore, the aim of the present study was to evaluate the cytotoxic effects of four calcium silicate-based cements on GDSC compared to that of intermediate restorative material (IRM; Caulk Dentsply, Midford, DE, USA). IRM is a commonly used temporary filling material that is highly toxic to human stem cells [18,20]; therefore, we used IRM as a negative control. We also evaluated the mineralization potential of the four calcium silicate-based cements on GDSCs.

2. Materials and Methods

2.1. Human Gingiva-Derived Stem Cells

GDSCs were collected using a previously reported method [21]. Gingival tissue was collected from a 70-year-old female undergoing a second implant surgery. The institutional review board of Seoul St. Mary's Hospital, College of Medicine, The Catholic University of Korea approved this study (KC19SESI0259), and written informed consent was obtained from the participant. All experiments were performed according to relevant guidelines and regulations specified in the Declaration of Helsinki.

Gingival tissue was de-epithelialized, minced into 1–2 mm^2 fragments, and digested in an alpha-modified minimal essential medium (α-MEM; Gibco, Grand Island, NY, USA) containing dispase (1 mg/mL; Sigma-Aldrich, St. Louis, MO, USA) and collagenase IV (2 mg/mL; Sigma-Aldrich). Cells were incubated in a humidified incubator at 37 °C. Every 2–3 days nonadherent cells were rinsed with phosphate-buffered saline (PBS; Welgene, Daegu, South Korea) and placed in fresh medium.

2.2. Experimental Disks of Four Calcium Silicate-Based Cements

The calcium silicate-based cements tested in the present study were ProRoot MTA (Dentsply Tulsa Dental Specialties), Biodentine (Septodont), Endocem Zr (Maruchi), and RetroMTA (BioMTA). Their compositions are presented in Table 1. All cements were mixed according to the manufacturer's guidelines. We produced disks of each cement 6 mm in diameter and 3 mm in height using sterile rubber molds under aseptic conditions. All disks were placed in a 100% humidity incubator at 37 °C for 48 h, then sterilized using ultraviolet light at room temperature for 4 h.

Table 1. The manufacturer and chemical composition of each experimental calcium silicate-based cement used in this study [17,22–24].

Material	Manufacturer	Composition	Batch Number
ProRoot MTA	Dentsply Tulsa Dental Specialties, Tulsa, OK, USA	Portland cement (tricalcium silicate, dicalcium silicate, and tricalcium aluminate) 75% Calcium sulfate dihydrate (gypsum) 5% Bismuth oxide 20%	0000186484
Biodentine	Septodont, Saint-Maur-des-Fossés, France	Tricalcium silicate, dicalcium silicate, calcium carbonate, calcium oxide, and zirconium oxide in its powder form Water, calcium chloride, and soluble polymer as an aqueous liquid	B24553
Endocem Zr	Maruchi, Wonju, Korea	Calcium oxide 27%–37% Silicon dioxide 7%–11% Aluminum oxide 3%–5% Magnesium oxide 1.7%–2.5% Ferrous oxide 1.3%–2.3% Zirconium dioxide 43%–46%	ZF7812231228
RetroMTA	BioMTA, Seoul, Korea	Calcium carbonate 60%–80% Silicon dioxide 5%–15% Aluminum oxide 5%–10% Calcium zirconia complex 20%–30%	RM1810D14

2.3. Cell Viability Assay

We evaluated the cytotoxic effects of the four calcium silicate-based cements using a methyl-thiazoldiphenyl-tetrazolium (MTT) assay (MTT Cell Growth Assay Kit; Chemicon, Rosemont, IL, USA) [25,26]. The proliferation rate of the GDSCs was analyzed after 0, 1, 2, 3, and 5 days of culture growth. GDSCs were seeded at a density of 1.0×10^4 cells/well on 24-well cell culture plates (SPL Life Sciences, Pocheon, Korea) with a growth medium. After 24 h of culture for cell attachment, we obtained the optical density value for day 0. An individual disk was stored in an insert with a 0.4 μm pore size (SPLInsert; SPL Life Sciences) and the insert was stored over the GDSCs. For maintaining the medium level up to the disk, each well was supplemented with an extra 1 mL of growth medium. GDSCs cultured without experimental disks were used as positive controls, and IRM was used as a negative control. MTT solution at a concentration of 500 μg/mL was added to each well for 4 h. Thereafter, each well was washed with PBS and dimethyl sulfoxide was added to dissolve the synthesized formazan. The optical density at 570 nm was determined using an absorbance microplate reader (Power Wave XS; BioTek Instruments, Winooski, VT, USA) with the absorbance at 630 nm as the reference. Each group was evaluated in quadruplicate.

2.4. Cell Migration Assay

We evaluated cell migratory ability using a scratch wound healing assay. GDSCs were seeded at a density of 3.5×10^4 cells/well on 24-well cell culture plates (SPL Life Sciences, Pocheon, Korea) with a growth medium. After 24 h of culture, a scratch wound was created in the middle of the confluent cell layer using a 1000 μL pipette tip. After scratching, cell debris was rinsed off with PBS. After 24 h of culture, each individual disk was stored in an insert with a 0.4 μm pore size (SPLInsert; SPL Life Sciences) and the insert was stored over the GDSCs. For maintaining the medium level up to the disk, each well was supplemented with an extra 1 mL of growth medium. GDSCs with various calcium silicate-based cement disks were incubated for 4 days, with changing the medium every 2 days. Images of wound healing were observed at 0, 1, 2, 3, and 4 days using a phase-contrast microscope (Olympus, Tokyo, Japan). ImageJ 1.46r (National Institutes of Health, Bethesda, MD, USA) was used to determine

2.5. Live/Dead Staining Assay

GDSCs were seeded at a density of 1.0×10^4 cells/well on 24-well plates (SPL Life Sciences) with a growth medium. After 24 h of culture, each individual disk was stored in an insert with a 0.4 μm pore size (SPLInsert; SPL Life Sciences) and the insert was stored over the GDSCs. GDSCs with various calcium silicate cement disks were incubated for 5 days, with changing the growth medium every 2 days. Cells were double-stained with a LIVE/DEAD™ Cell Imaging Kit (488/570; Molecular Probes, Life Technologies, CA, USA) on days 3 and 5, and the stained cells were evaluated under an inverted microscope (Axiovert 200; Carl Zeiss Microscopy, Jena, Germany). Qualitative analyses of cell viability were performed with digital image processing software (ZEN 2012, AxioVision; Carl Zeiss Microscopy).

2.6. Alizarin Red S (ARS) Staining Assay

To evaluate the formation of calcified nodules in GDSCs, we used an ARS assay [25,26]. The powder of each experimental calcium silicate-based cement was mixed with an osteogenic medium at a concentration of 5 mg/mL, and the mixture was placed in a 100% humidity incubator at 37 °C for 7 days. The osteogenic medium consisted of complete α-MEM, 50 μg/mL ascorbic acid (Sigma-Aldrich), 0.1 μM dexamethasone (Sigma-Aldrich), and 10 mM beta-glycerophosphate (Sigma-Aldrich). The supernatant fluid was refined through 0.20 μm filters (Minisart; Sartorius Stedim Biotech, Goetingen, Germany). GDSCs were seeded at a density of 2.0×10^4 cells/well on 24-well plates (SPL Life Sciences) and cultured for 21 days in calcium silicate-based cement eluate, with changing the eluate every 3 days. Cells were fixed in 4% paraformaldehyde solution and stained with 2% ARS solution (ScienCell, Carlsbad, CA, USA) for 20 min. The stain was treated with 10% cetylpyridinium chloride (Sigma-Aldrich) for 15 min, and the optical density at 560 nm was evaluated using an absorbance microplate reader (Power Wave XS). Each group was evaluated in quadruplicate.

2.7. pH Measurement

The powder of each experimental calcium silicate-based cement was mixed with deionized water and osteogenic medium at a concentration of 5 mg/mL, and the mixture was placed in a 100% humidity incubator at 37 °C for 7 days. The pH of each liquid was evaluated using a digital pH meter which is adjusted prior calibration (Satorious Docu-pH Meter; Satorious AG, Goettingen, Germany). Three measurements were made for each cement solution. As a control, deionized water and osteogenic medium without experimental powder was also measured.

2.8. Statistical Analyses

The SPSS software program (ver. 24.0; IBM Corp., Armonk, NY, USA) was used for statistical analyses. The Shapiro-Wilk test of normality was used to confirm the data distribution. The data normality was confirmed; thus, repeated measures analyses of variance were performed for general comparisons of MTT and wound healing assays. Independent *t* tests were performed for pairwise comparisons of experimental groups at each time point. One-way analyses of variance and Tukey *post hoc* tests were used for the ARS assay. $p < 0.05$ was considered statistically significant.

3. Results

In the cell viability assay, no significant differences were shown among the ProRoot MTA, Biodentine, and positive control groups during the test period ($p > 0.05$). The Endocem Zr and RetroMTA groups differed significantly from the control group on days 5 and 7 ($p < 0.05$). Out of all groups, the IRM group showed the lowest viable cell level after 24 h ($p < 0.05$) (Figure 1).

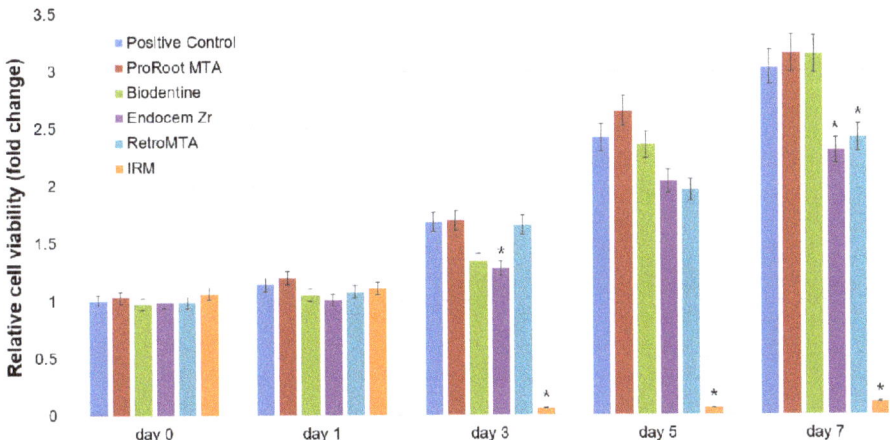

Figure 1. Relative cell viability based on methyl-thiazoldiphenyl-tetrazolium (MTT) assay. Asterisks represent statistically significant differences between the positive control and experimental groups.

In the cell migration assay, no significant differences were found among the ProRoot MTA, Biodentine, Endocem Zr, and control groups during the test period ($p > 0.05$). The RetroMTA group had lower cell migratory ability than the control group on days 3 and 4 ($p < 0.05$). Cell migration was not shown in the IRM group, and significant differences were observed between the IRM and positive control groups at days 1–4 ($p < 0.05$; Figure 2). Representative images of the cell migration in all groups are shown in Figure 3.

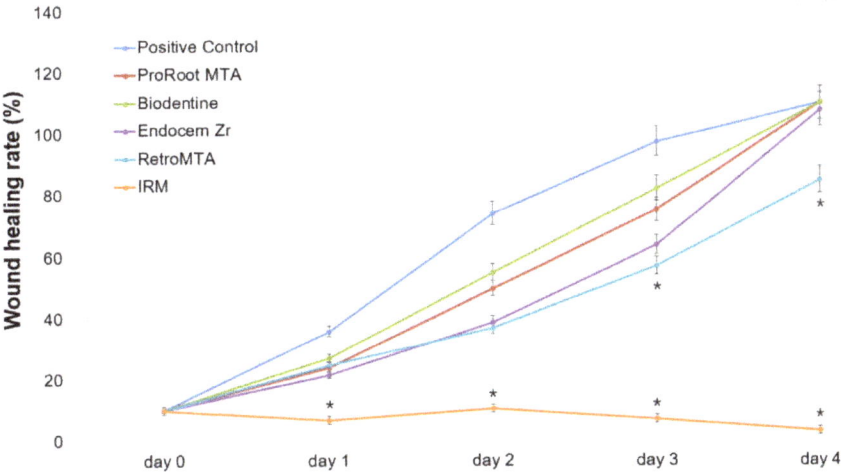

Figure 2. Wound healing rate of all tested calcium silicate-based cements. Asterisks represent statistically significant differences between the positive control and experimental groups.

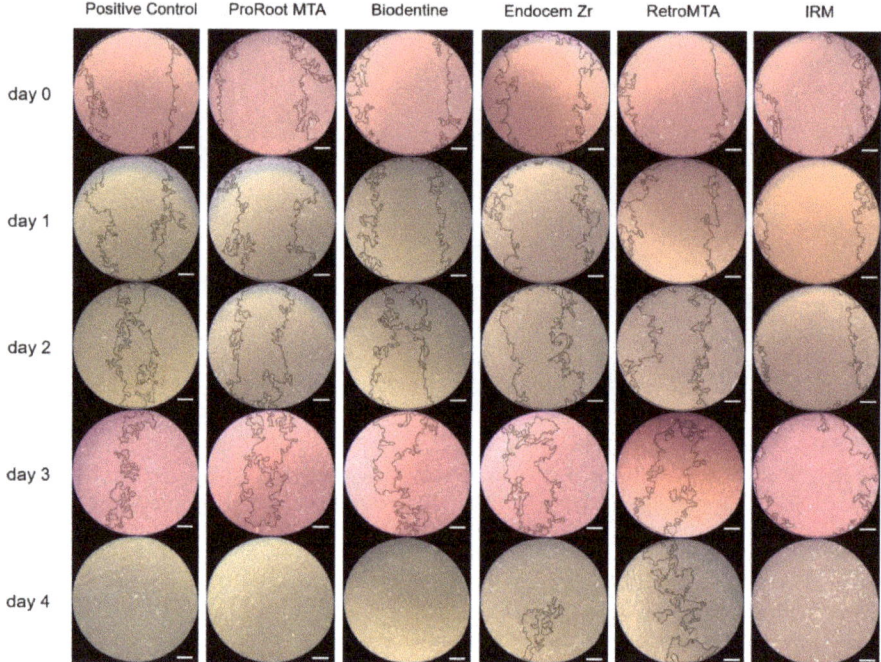

Figure 3. Representative images of cell migration based on wound healing assay (scale bar = 250 μm).

In the live/dead staining assay, GDSCs in contact with IRM extract showed low viable cell density, whereas GDSCs in contact with the other experimental cements showed favorable cell growth relative to the control group (Figure 4).

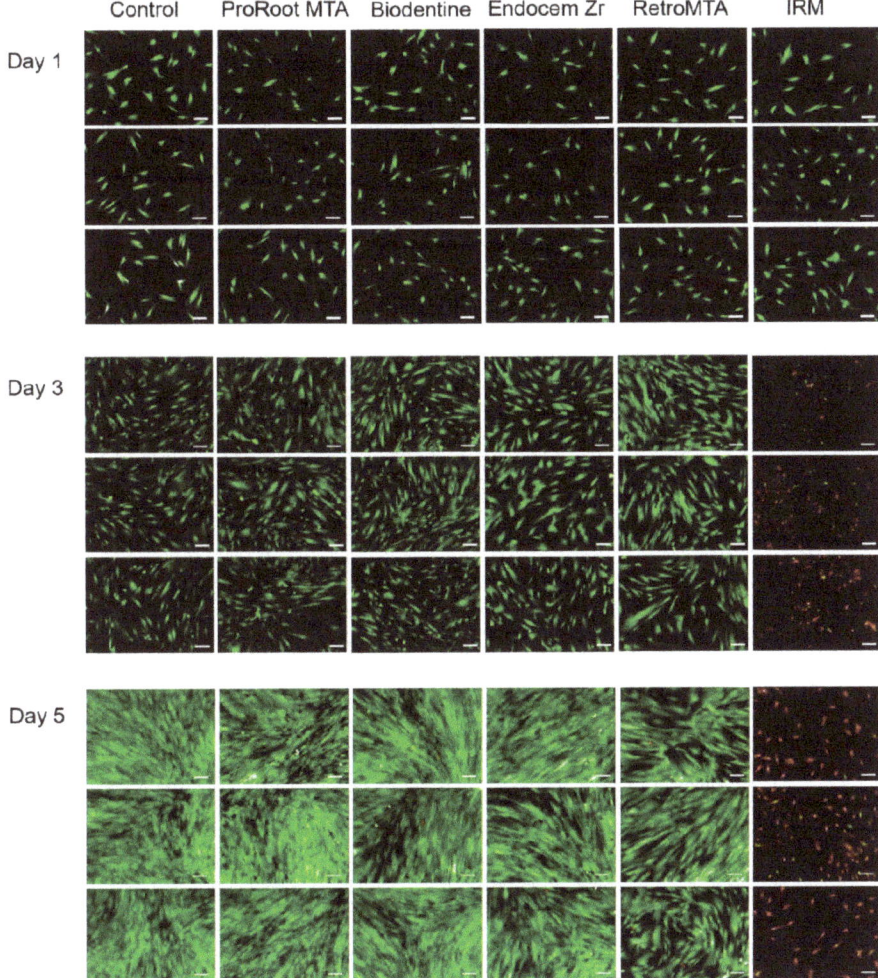

Figure 4. Results of live/dead staining assay of all tested calcium silicate-based cements (scale bar = 200 μm).

In the ARS assay, GDSCs exposed to ProRoot MTA, Biodentine, and RetroMTA eluates resulted in a meaningful increase in the formation of calcium (Ca) compared to the Endocem Zr and control groups on day 21 ($p < 0.05$; Figure 5).

In the pH measurement, the pH of all experimental calcium silicate-based cements in deionized water was higher (pH > 10.0) than the pH of deionized water without experimental powder (Table 2).

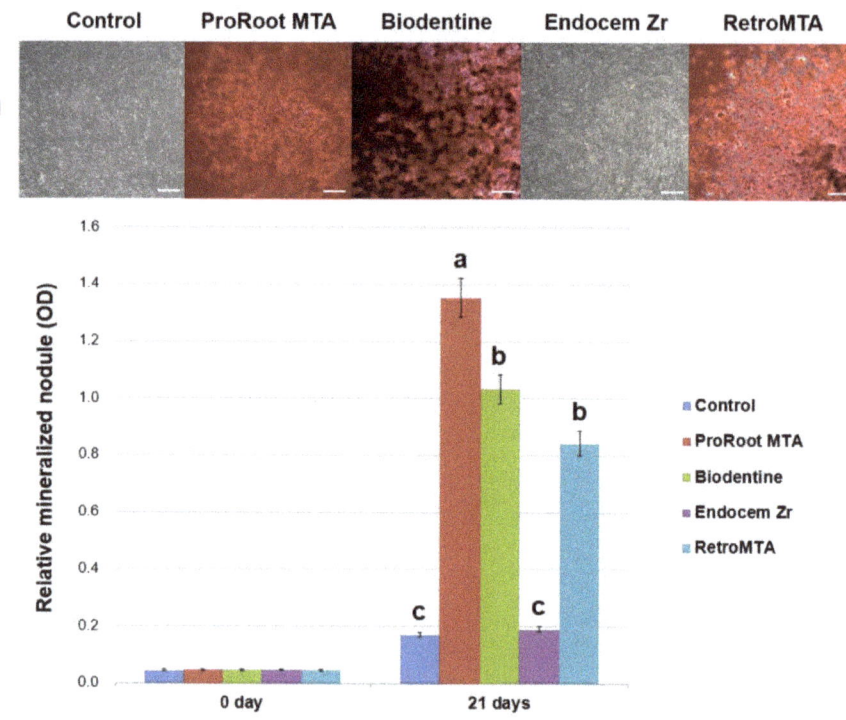

Figure 5. Relative rate of mineralized nodule formation based on Alizarin red staining assay. Different superscript letters indicate statistically significant differences (scale bar = 500 μm).

Table 2. The pH of each experimental calcium silicate-based cement.

Material	pH (7 days)							
	Osteogenic Media				ddH_2O			
				Mean				Mean
Control	7.56	7.59	7.50	**7.55**	7.02	7.06	7.08	**7.05**
ProRoot MTA	8.58	8.63	8.67	**8.63**	11.33	11.34	11.29	**11.32**
Biodentine	9.65	9.71	9.67	**9.68**	11.31	11.30	11.34	**11.32**
Endocem Zr	8.61	8.69	8.74	**8.68**	10.77	10.79	10.82	**10.79**
RetroMTA	8.55	8.57	8.58	**8.57**	11.32	11.35	11.32	**11.33**

4. Discussion

In some clinical conditions such as the repair of root resorption, a fast initial setting time is required to prevent the dissolution of materials into blood and oral fluids. Less tooth discoloration is also an important factor esthetically. Some alternative calcium silicate-based cements, such as Biodentine, Endocem Zr, and RetroMTA, were introduced for these reasons to replace ProRoot MTA. Furthermore, biocompatible and bioactive calcium silicate-based cements can promote rapid healing of adjacent periodontal tissue. Therefore, in the present study we evaluated the cytotoxicity and mineralization potential of four calcium silicate-based cements on GDSCs.

In this study, we analyzed the biocompatibility of ProRoot MTA, Biodentine, Endocem Zr, RetroMTA, and IRM using MTT and wound healing assays. The ProRoot MTA, Biodentine, and control groups showed higher cell viability and migratory ability compared to the IRM group. The Endocem

Zr and RetroMTA groups showed lower cell viability compared to the control group (Figure 1), and the RetroMTA group also had a slower cell migration rate than the control group (Figure 2).

Biodentine is a novel bioceramic calcium silicate-based cement that possesses biocompatible and noncytotoxic properties [22,27]. In one study, the highest migration rate of dental pulp stem cells was found in the Biodentine group, and scanning electron microscopy revealed superior cell adhesion on disks of Biodentine [22]. In another study, cell viability was highest in the Biodentine group followed by the ProRoot MTA group, although viability on the glass ionomer cement (Ketac Molar Aplicap; 3M ESPE, Seefeld, Germany) was significantly lower [27]. Other published studies showed that Biodentine eluates resulted in low-to-moderate negative consequence on cell viability and on cell migratory ability [28]. One possible explanation is that high density level of Biodentine in the growth medium seriously lower stem cell proliferation [29].

Endocem Zr is a pozzolan-based, white calcium silicate cement developed to improve shortcomings such as a long setting time and tooth discoloration [30]. If bismuth oxide, which is used as a radiopacifier in ProRoot MTA, interacts with the collagen fibrils in dentin, it can lead to tooth discoloration. Bismuth oxide is substituted by zirconium oxide in the Endocem Zr formulation [31]. Lee et al. reported that Endocem Zr showed a similar inflammatory response to dental pulp tissue as did ProRoot MTA; however, its formation of a calcific barrier was inferior to that by ProRoot MTA [30].

RetroMTA is another fast-setting calcium silicate cement thanks to its zirconium component, which shortens the setting time by increasing the hydration rate of Portland cement [32]. In a study by Chung et al., RetroMTA showed similar biocompatibility and angiogenic effects on human dental pulp cells as ProRoot MTA; therefore, it is an effective pulp capping material [33]. In comparison, Endocem Zr showed irregular cytotoxic effects and derived less vascular endothelial growth factor and angiogenin expression [33]. In a previous study, both ProRoot MTA and RetroMTA resulted in significantly higher cell viability compared to the positive control, whereas ProRoot MTA had a higher radiopacity than RetroMTA [23]. Another study found that set RetroMTA showed better biological responses compared to a set calcium-enriched mixture (BioniqueDent, Tehran, Iran) and Angelus MTA (Angelus MTA, Londrina, Paraná, Brazil) in a mouse L929 fibroblast cell line [19].

In this study, we evaluated the calcium nodule formation ability associated with ProRoot MTA, Biodentine, Endocem Zr, and RetroMTA using an ARS assay. We found that ProRoot MTA resulted in more mineralization potential than Biodentine and RetroMTA, which is in accordance with a previous study in which ProRoot MTA showed better osteogenic potential than Biodentine based on real-time polymerase chain reaction expression analysis, alkaline phosphatase activity, and calcium nodule formation data [34]. In another study, Biodentine showed significantly decreased alkaline phosphatase activity compared to ProRoot MTA [35]. Its differences in composition and the rate of dissolution in culture medium may be one reason for the lower mineralization activity of Biodentine [34]. Differences in types of cells, culture condition, and time of culturing may have affected the results. In both studies, alveolar bone marrow stem cells rather than dental pulp stem cells were used [34,35].

Meanwhile, a different study showed that Biodentine has a comparable efficacy to ProRoot MTA in the clinical setting and may be considered as an interesting substitute for ProRoot MTA in pulp capping procedures [36]. In that study, well-arranged odontoblast layers and odontoblast-like cells formed tubular dentin under the osteodentin [36]. Furthermore, Wongwatanasanti et al. reported that only Biodentine showed a positive ARS compared to ProRoot MTA and RetroMTA groups [37]. They concluded that Biodentine, ProRoot MTA, and RetroMTA all induce stem cell apical papilla (SCAP) proliferation; however, only Biodentine induces significant SCAP differentiation [37]. Another study also showed that SCAP mineralization was greater in the Biodentine group than the ProRoot MTA group [38]. These studies used SCAP for the ARS assay [37,38], unlike our study, which used GDSCs. The differences in osteogenic gene expression can be explained by differences in cell origin and developmental status at the time of incubation. Therefore, further investigation is required to clarify the different results.

A previous study reported that Endocem MTA and Endocem Zr are related with remarkably less Ca ion release compared to ProRoot MTA [31]. When the three cements were immersed in PBS for 2 weeks, these cements created Ca- and phosphorous (P)-incorporating apatite-like materials. ProRoot MTA showed precipitates which has a higher Ca/P ratio compared to Endocem Zr [31]. Unlike ProRoot MTA, in which calcium and silicon are the predominant compositions, Endocem Zr is largely composed of zirconia with a small quantity of calcium and silicon. In the present study, Endocem Zr showed the lowest calcium nodule formation ability among the experimental calcium silicate-based cements, in accordance with a previous study [30]. Ca ions contribute to the formation and mineralization of hard tissue. Therefore, extended Ca release from calcium silicate-based cements can influence the osteogenic potential of bone marrow stem cells and osteoblast progenitors [39,40]. In the present study, all tested calcium silicate-based cements were associated with an alkaline pH (Table 2), consistent with the findings of previous studies [23,41,42]. The high alkalinity of the materials contributes to their osteogenic potential as a suitable condition for matrix formation and antimicrobial ability is created.

Unfortunately, the reason why various calcium silicate-based cements elicit different biological responses was not thoroughly investigated in this study. Further study on the association between chemical components of the calcium silicate-based cements and biological responses of cells is necessary. Furthermore, proper characterization of each calcium silicate-based cement is required.

5. Conclusions

In summary, the four calcium silicate-based cements evaluated in this study using GDSCs had good biological properties. The ProRoot MTA, Biodentine, and RetroMTA groups showed higher mineralization potential compared to the Endocem Zr and control groups. Therefore, Biodentine and RetroMTA can be used as alternatives to ProRoot MTA to treat ERR in terms of esthetics. Further in vivo research is needed.

Author Contributions: D.L. and J.-B.P. contributed equally to this work. D.L., J.-B.P., and S.-Y.K. participated in the conceptualization and design of the study. D.L., D.S., and H.-M.K. performed all the experimental procedures and contributed to data acquisition. D.L., J.-B.P., D.S., H.-M.K. and S.-Y.K. contributed substantially to data interpretation and analysis. D.L., J.-B.P., and S.-Y.K. were involved in drafting the manuscript and revising it critically for important intellectual content. All authors have read and agreed to the published version of the manuscript.

Funding: This research was funded by a National Research Foundation of Korea (NRF) grant funded by the Korean government (Ministry of Science, ICT and Future Planning) (no. 2017R1C1B5017098 and 2019R1F1A1058955).

Conflicts of Interest: The authors declare no conflicts of interest.

References

1. Fuss, Z.; Tsesis, I.; Lin, S. Root resorption—Diagnosis, classification and treatment choices based on stimulation factors. *Dent. Traumatol.* **2003**, *19*, 175–182. [CrossRef]
2. Heithersay, G.S. Management of tooth resorption. *Aust. Dent. J.* **2007**, *52*, S105–S121. [CrossRef]
3. Karypidou, A.; Chatzinikolaou, I.D.; Kouros, P.; Koulaouzidou, E.; Economides, N. Management of bilateral invasive cervical resorption lesions in maxillary incisors using a novel calcium silicate-based cement: A case report. *Quintessence Int.* **2016**, *47*, 637–642. [CrossRef]
4. Duarte, M.A.H.; Marciano, M.A.; Vivan, R.R.; Tanomaru Filho, M.; Tanomaru, J.M.G.; Camilleri, J. Tricalcium silicate-based cements: Properties and modifications. *Braz. Oral Res.* **2018**, *32*, e70. [CrossRef]
5. Camilleri, J. Characterization and hydration kinetics of tricalcium silicate cement for use as a dental biomaterial. *Dent. Mater.* **2011**, *27*, 836–844. [CrossRef]
6. Torabinejad, M.; Parirokh, M.; Dummer, P.M.H. Mineral trioxide aggregate and other bioactive endodontic cements: An updated overview—Part II: Other clinical applications and complications. *Int. Endod. J.* **2018**, *51*, 284–317. [CrossRef]
7. Peng, W.; Liu, W.; Zhai, W.; Jiang, L.; Li, L.; Chang, J.; Zhu, Y. Effect of tricalcium silicate on the proliferation and odontogenic differentiation of human dental pulp cells. *J. Endod.* **2011**, *37*, 1240–1246. [CrossRef]

8. Du, R.; Wu, T.; Liu, W.; Li, L.; Jiang, L.; Peng, W.; Chang, J.; Zhu, Y. Role of the extracellular signal-regulated kinase 1/2 pathway in driving tricalcium silicate-induced proliferation and biomineralization of human dental pulp cells in vitro. *J. Endod.* **2013**, *39*, 1023–1029. [CrossRef]
9. Rathinam, E.; Rajasekharan, S.; Chitturi, R.T.; Martens, L.; De Coster, P. Gene expression profiling and molecular signaling of dental pulp cells in response to tricalcium silicate cements: A systematic review. *J. Endod.* **2015**, *41*, 1805–1817. [CrossRef]
10. Marciano, M.A.; Camilleri, J.; Costa, R.M.; Matsumoto, M.A.; Guimaraes, B.M.; Duarte, M.A.H. Zinc oxide inhibits dental discoloration caused by white mineral trioxide aggregate Angelus. *J. Endod.* **2017**, *43*, 1001–1007. [CrossRef]
11. Dawood, A.E.; Parashos, P.; Wong, R.H.K.; Reynolds, E.C.; Manton, D.J. Calcium silicate-based cements: Composition, properties, and clinical applications. *J. Investig. Clin. Dent.* **2017**, *8*. [CrossRef] [PubMed]
12. Loison-Robert, L.S.; Tassin, M.; Bonte, E.; Berbar, T.; Isaac, J.; Berdal, A.; Simon, S.; Fournier, B.P.J. In vitro effects of two silicate-based materials, Biodentine and BioRoot RCS, on dental pulp stem cells in models of reactionary and reparative dentinogenesis. *PLoS ONE* **2018**, *13*, e0190014. [CrossRef] [PubMed]
13. Li, Q.; Hurt, A.P.; Coleman, N.J. The application of (29)Si NMR spectroscopy to the analysis of calcium silicate-based cement using Biodentine™ as an example. *J. Funct. Biomater.* **2019**, *10*, 25. [CrossRef]
14. Setbon, H.M.; Devaux, J.; Iserentant, A.; Leloup, G.; Leprince, J.G. Influence of composition on setting kinetics of new injectable and/or fast setting tricalcium silicate cements. *Dent. Mater.* **2014**, *30*, 1291–1303. [CrossRef] [PubMed]
15. Camilleri, J.; Laurent, P.; About, I. Hydration of Biodentine, Theracal LC, and a prototype tricalcium silicate-based dentin replacement material after pulp capping in entire tooth cultures. *J. Endod.* **2014**, *40*, 1846–1854. [CrossRef] [PubMed]
16. Zanini, M.; Sautier, J.M.; Berdal, A.; Simon, S. Biodentine induces immortalized murine pulp cell differentiation into odontoblast-like cells and stimulates biomineralization. *J. Endod.* **2012**, *38*, 1220–1226. [CrossRef] [PubMed]
17. Kang, S.H.; Shin, Y.S.; Lee, H.S.; Kim, S.O.; Shin, Y.; Jung, I.Y.; Song, J.S. Color changes of teeth after treatment with various mineral trioxide aggregate-based materials: An ex vivo study. *J. Endod.* **2015**, *41*, 737–741. [CrossRef]
18. Choi, Y.; Park, S.J.; Lee, S.H.; Hwang, Y.C.; Yu, M.K.; Min, K.S. Biological effects and washout resistance of a newly developed fast-setting pozzolan cement. *J. Endod.* **2013**, *39*, 467–472. [CrossRef]
19. Pornamazeh, T.; Yadegari, Z.; Ghasemi, A.; Sheykh-Al-Eslamian, S.M.; Shojaeian, S. In vitro cytotoxicity and setting time assessment of calcium-enriched mixture cement, Retro mineral trioxide aggregate and mineral trioxide aggregate. *Iran. Endod. J.* **2017**, *12*, 488–492. [CrossRef]
20. Collado-Gonzalez, M.; Garcia-Bernal, D.; Onate-Sanchez, R.E.; Ortolani-Seltenerich, P.S.; Alvarez-Muro, T.; Lozano, A.; Forner, L.; Llena, C.; Moraleda, J.M.; Rodriguez-Lozano, F.J. Cytotoxicity and bioactivity of various pulpotomy materials on stem cells from human exfoliated primary teeth. *Int. Endod. J.* **2017**, *50*, e19–e30. [CrossRef]
21. Jin, S.H.; Lee, J.E.; Yun, J.H.; Kim, I.; Ko, Y.; Park, J.B. Isolation and characterization of human mesenchymal stem cells from gingival connective tissue. *J. Periodontal Res.* **2015**, *50*, 461–467. [CrossRef] [PubMed]
22. Tomás-Catalá, C.J.; Collado-González, M.; García-Bernal, D.; Oñate-Sánchez, R.E.; Forner, L.; Llena, C.; Lozano, A.; Moraleda, J.M.; Rodríguez-Lozano, F.J. Biocompatibility of new pulp-capping materials NeoMTA Plus, MTA Repair HP, and Biodentine on human dental pulp stem cells. *J. Endod.* **2018**, *44*, 126–132. [CrossRef] [PubMed]
23. Souza, L.C.D.; Yadlapati, M.; Dorn, S.O.; Silva, R.; Letra, A. Analysis of radiopacity, pH and cytotoxicity of a new bioceramic material. *J. Appl. Oral Sci.* **2015**, *23*, 383–389. [CrossRef] [PubMed]
24. Youssef, A.R.; Emara, R.; Taher, M.M.; Al-Allaf, F.A.; Almalki, M.; Almasri, M.A.; Siddiqui, S.S. Effects of mineral trioxide aggregate, calcium hydroxide, Biodentine and Emdogain on osteogenesis, odontogenesis, angiogenesis and cell viability of dental pulp stem cells. *BMC Oral Health* **2019**, *19*, 133. [CrossRef]
25. Kim, H.S.; Zheng, M.; Kim, D.K.; Lee, W.P.; Yu, S.J.; Kim, B.O. Effects of 1,25-dihydroxyvitamin D3 on the differentiation of MC3T3-E1 osteoblast-like cells. *J. Periodontal Implant Sci.* **2018**, *48*, 34–46. [CrossRef]
26. Hwang, J.H.; Oh, S.; Kim, S. Improvement of the osteogenic potential of ErhBMP-2-/EGCG-coated biphasic calcium phosphate bone substitute: In vitro and in vivo activity. *J. Periodontal Implant Sci.* **2019**, *49*, 114–126. [CrossRef]

27. Widbiller, M.; Lindner, S.R.; Buchalla, W.; Eidt, A.; Hiller, K.A.; Schmalz, G.; Galler, K.M. Three-dimensional culture of dental pulp stem cells in direct contact to tricalcium silicate cements. *Clin. Oral Investig.* **2016**, *20*, 237–246. [CrossRef]
28. Sequeira, D.B.; Seabra, C.M.; Palma, P.J.; Cardoso, A.L.; Peça, J.; Santos, J.M. Effects of a new bioceramic material on human apical papilla cells. *J. Funct. Biomater.* **2018**, *9*, 74. [CrossRef]
29. Luo, Z.; Li, D.; Kohli, M.R.; Yu, Q.; Kim, S.; He, W.-X. Effect of Biodentine™ on the proliferation, migration and adhesion of human dental pulp stem cells. *J. Dent.* **2014**, *42*, 490–497. [CrossRef]
30. Lee, M.; Kang, C.M.; Song, J.S.; Shin, Y.; Kim, S.; Kim, S.O.; Choi, H.J. Biological efficacy of two mineral trioxide aggregate (MTA)-based materials in a canine model of pulpotomy. *Dent. Mater. J.* **2017**, *36*, 41–47. [CrossRef]
31. Han, L.; Kodama, S.; Okiji, T. Evaluation of calcium-releasing and apatite-forming abilities of fast-setting calcium silicate-based endodontic materials. *Int. Endod. J.* **2015**, *48*, 124–130. [CrossRef] [PubMed]
32. Li, Q.; Deacon, A.D.; Coleman, N.J. The impact of zirconium oxide nanoparticles on the hydration chemistry and biocompatibility of white Portland cement. *Dent. Mater. J.* **2013**, *32*, 808–815. [CrossRef] [PubMed]
33. Chung, C.J.; Kim, E.; Song, M.; Park, J.W.; Shin, S.J. Effects of two fast-setting calcium-silicate cements on cell viability and angiogenic factor release in human pulp-derived cells. *Odontology* **2016**, *104*, 143–151. [CrossRef]
34. Margunato, S.; Tasli, P.N.; Aydin, S.; Karapinar Kazandag, M.; Sahin, F. In vitro evaluation of ProRoot MTA, Biodentine, and MM-MTA on human alveolar bone marrow stem cells in terms of biocompatibility and mineralization. *J. Endod.* **2015**, *41*, 1646–1652. [CrossRef] [PubMed]
35. Sultana, N.; Singh, M.; Nawal, R.R.; Chaudhry, S.; Yadav, S.; Mohanty, S.; Talwar, S. Evaluation of biocompatibility and osteogenic potential of tricalcium silicate-based cements using human bone marrow-derived mesenchymal stem cells. *J. Endod.* **2018**, *44*, 446–451. [CrossRef]
36. Nowicka, A.; Lipski, M.; Parafiniuk, M.; Sporniak-Tutak, K.; Lichota, D.; Kosierkiewicz, A.; Kaczmarek, W.; Buczkowska-Radlinska, J. Response of human dental pulp capped with biodentine and mineral trioxide aggregate. *J. Endod.* **2013**, *39*, 743–747. [CrossRef] [PubMed]
37. Wongwatanasanti, N.; Jantarat, J.; Sritanaudomchai, H.; Hargreaves, K.M. Effect of bioceramic materials on proliferation and odontoblast differentiation of human stem cells from the apical papilla. *J. Endod.* **2018**, *44*, 1270–1275. [CrossRef]
38. Wattanapakkavong, K.; Srisuwan, T. Release of transforming growth factor beta 1 from human tooth dentin after application of either ProRoot MTA or Biodentine as a coronal barrier. *J. Endod.* **2019**, *45*, 701–705. [CrossRef]
39. Khan, S.; Kaleem, M.; Fareed, M.A.; Habib, A.; Iqbal, K.; Aslam, A.; Ud Din, S. Chemical and morphological characteristics of mineral trioxide aggregate and Portland cements. *Dent. Mater. J.* **2016**, *35*, 112–117. [CrossRef]
40. Formosa, L.M.; Mallia, B.; Bull, T.; Camilleri, J. The microstructure and surface morphology of radiopaque tricalcium silicate cement exposed to different curing conditions. *Dent. Mater.* **2012**, *28*, 584–595. [CrossRef]
41. Kim, M.; Yang, W.; Kim, H.; Ko, H. Comparison of the biological properties of ProRoot MTA, OrthoMTA, and Endocem MTA cements. *J. Endod.* **2014**, *40*, 1649–1653. [CrossRef] [PubMed]
42. Parirokh, M.; Torabinejad, M. Mineral trioxide aggregate: A comprehensive literature review—Part I: Chemical, physical, and antibacterial properties. *J. Endod.* **2010**, *36*, 16–27. [CrossRef] [PubMed]

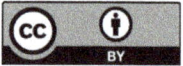

© 2020 by the authors. Licensee MDPI, Basel, Switzerland. This article is an open access article distributed under the terms and conditions of the Creative Commons Attribution (CC BY) license (http://creativecommons.org/licenses/by/4.0/).

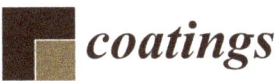

Article

Calcium Sulfate in Implantology (Biphasic Calcium Sul-Fate/Hydroxyapatite, BCS/HA, Bond Apatite®): Review of the Literature and Case Reports

Aina Torrejon-Moya [1], Alina Apalimova [1], Beatriz González-Navarro [1], Ramiro Zaera-Le Gal [2], Antonio Marí-Roig [3] and José López-López [4,*]

1. Faculty of Medicine and Health Sciences (Dentistry), University of Barcelona, 08907 L'Hospitalet de Llobregat, Spain
2. Private Practice, 08029 Barcelona, Spain
3. Department of Maxillofacial Surgery, Bellvitge University Hospital, 08907 L'Hospitalet de Llobregrat, Spain
4. Department of Oral Medicine, Oral Surgery and Oral Implantology, Faculty of Dentistry, Service of the Medical-Surgical Area of Dentistry Hospital, University of Barcelona, 08907 L'Hospitalet de Llobregat, Spain
* Correspondence: jl.lopez@ub.edu

Abstract: Calcium sulfate is used as a synthetic graft material in orthopedics, plastic surgery, oncological surgery, and dentistry, and it has been used in a variety of clinical applications, such as the repair of periodontal defects, the treatment of osteomyelitis, maxillary sinus augmentation, and as a complement to the placement of dental implants. To carry out this systematic review, a bibliographic search was carried out. The PICO (Patient, Intervention, Comparison, Outcome) question was: Does the use of calcium sulfate as a material in guided bone regeneration in dentistry have better results compared to other bone graft materials? Finally, a case series is presented using the calcium sulfate for different procedures. Currently, the available literature on the use of calcium sulfate as a graft material in implant surgery is scarce, and what is available provides low-quality evidence. That is why more research studies on the subject are necessary to allow more comparisons and meaningful conclusions. After using Bond Apatite® in our case series, we can conclude that it is a useful and easy-to-handle material in implantology practice, but more controlled studies should be carried out in this regard to assess its long-term efficacy, especially in horizontal and/or vertical regeneration.

Keywords: calcium sulfate; dental implant; guided bone regeneration; sinus lift

1. Introduction

The use of dental implants has become a common treatment modality and an important component of modern dentistry [1]. In many clinical situations, the edentulous areas to be rehabilitated do not offer adequate bone volume for implant placement; this may be due to different causes, such as the presence of anatomical structures that limit it (maxillary sinuses, presence of nerves or vessels, etc.) due to early bone atrophy and the traumatic extraction of a tooth or periodontal disease [2,3]. Tooth extraction is associated with the remodeling of the alveolar process and results in changes, both structural and dimensional, with horizontal losses of up to 29%–63% and vertical losses of 11%–22% at 6 months after tooth extraction [4,5].

For such defects, guided bone regeneration procedures before or in combination with implant placement are necessary [6]. These procedures are based on the use of different types of graft materials and membranes. The bone substitute must be osteoconductive, to act as a scaffold maintaining three-dimensional support during bone healing, and also osteoinductive, stimulating bone formation; the membranes act as a barrier and seal the area to be regenerated to prevent the ingrowth of soft tissue [7,8].

Historically, the most widely used grafting material was autologous bone, both extraoral and intraoral [9,10]; however, obtaining autogenous bone has several negative aspects, such as increased morbidity for the patient, limited supply, and increased duration of the intervention [11,12].

We currently have different types of bone graft materials for dental applications. Depending on the origin, they are classified as autografts, allografts, xenografts, or alloplastic grafts and can be found in the form of granules, putties, gels, and pastes, or blocks [13].

One of these alloplastic grafts is calcium sulfate, which is a common bone substitute and with a history of clinical use spanning more than 100 years, the first report of its use as a bone graft material was by the German physician Dreesman in 1892 when it was used as a treatment to seal bone defects in the long bones of eight patients with tuberculosis, according to Pelteier et al., in their work from 1957 [14]. This material is highly biocompatible and osteoconductive, undergoing practically complete resorption in vivo, and can be used as a vehicle to administer antibiotics, pharmacological agents, and growth factors [14,15].

Therefore, calcium sulfate, which is a bioactive material that produces the release of abundant calcium ions, is used as a synthetic graft material in orthopedics, plastic surgery, oncological surgery, and dentistry, and it has been used in a variety of clinical applications, such as the repair of periodontal defects, the treatment of osteomyelitis, and maxillary sinus augmentation, and as a complement to the placement of dental implants [16–19].

However, despite its many indications, it has some deficiencies that have prevented its daily use in dentistry, highlighting its rapid and complete resorption and hardening difficulties in the presence of saliva and bleeding. In 2010, Dr. Amos Yahav presented Bond Apatite® (Augma Biomaterials Ltd., Caesara Industrial Park, Israel & Microdent, Santa Eulàlia de Ronçana, Barcelona, Spain), a biphasic calcium sulfate that has proven to be more stable and with better properties than classic calcium sulfate [20,21]. It is a bone graft material composed of 2/3 biphasic calcium sulfate and 1/3 synthetic hydroxyapatite of different granulometry. Being the only one available, it is made of calcium sulfate and having the addition of hydroxyapatite. Calcium sulfate is reabsorbed and it is the hydroxyapatite particles that maintain volume during the process of new bone formation [22–24].

According to the study carried out by Yahav et al. [24], the addition of HA prolongs the resorption time and remains within the practical timeframe for dental clinical applications; most of the graft material is converted into young bone within 3 to 6 months, and the remainder is resorbed shortly thereafter.

Recent studies [19,20] have demonstrated successful results in guided bone regeneration with the use of calcium sulfate, and in addition, based on histological analysis, the percentage of graft remaining was relatively low, with no evidence of inflammatory response or graft encapsulation.

In this preparation, there are several considerations of interest. In the first place, thanks to the Biphasic Calcium Sulfate formulation (hemihydrated/dihydrated), the setting process can be reduced from about 20 min to 3, facilitating clinical management. In addition, the synthetic hydroxyapatite particles decrease the rate of graft resorption, maintaining volume; the smaller ones (90 microns) are reabsorbed after 3–4 months and the larger ones (1 mm), which represent 10% of the total hydroxyapatite, are reabsorbed after 8 months. Finally, the high porosity of the product, greater than 46%, favors the infiltration of growth factors, osteoblasts, and angiogenesis [15,25,26].

Whereas with conventional graft materials there is integration with the graft particles resulting in 20%–25% vital bone formation, with Bond Apatite®, there is no integration between the newly formed bone, and the material is completely resorbed. Instead, new vital bone is formed at the end of the regeneration process.

Biphasic calcium sulfate serves as a cement, and its rigid structure after a quick setting prevents epithelial–conjunctive cell infiltration into the material, acting as a barrier membrane. However, connective cells can multiply on the material's surface, encouraging the rapid repair of the overlying soft tissue [24].

Bond Apatite® is presented as a powder in a double barrel syringe and a sodium chloride solution. With the help of a piston, the solution is poured over the powder, obtaining a mixture that can be easily deposited in the bone deficit, since the resulting product is adhesive. Subsequently, pressure must be exerted with a dry sterile gauze for a few seconds, thus eliminating excess liquid and favoring the setting of the product. In addition, the manufacturer recommends closing the flap under tension and it is not necessary to cover the graft with any type of membrane, since when it hardens it acts as a barrier preventing the penetration of epithelial–connective cells [25,26].

This study aims to review the existing literature on calcium sulfate in oral surgery and expose various clinical cases using Bond Apatite® as a bone graft material in different situations. Therefore, the following PICO (Patient, Intervention, Comparison, Outcome) question was: Does the use of calcium sulfate as a material in guided bone regeneration in dentistry have better results compared to other bone graft materials?

2. Materials and Methods

To carry out this systematic review, a bibliographic search was carried out in the MEDLINE database through PubMed.

The following combinations of keywords were performed: "calcium sulfate" [MeSH Terms] AND ("surgery, oral" [MeSH Terms] OR "oral surgical procedures" [MeSH Terms]), "calcium sulfate" [MeSH Terms] AND "bone regeneration" [MeSH Terms], (calcium sulfate [MeSH Terms]) AND (bone grafting [MeSH Terms]).

The articles that were included in this systematic review had to meet the following inclusion criteria: controlled clinical trials, randomized controlled clinical trials, and case series, with more than 30 participants, carried out in humans and published within the last 10 years in English. Studies outside the field of dentistry, systematic reviews, preclinical studies, and clinical trials with insufficient information were excluded.

Finally, a case series is presented using the calcium sulfate for different procedures. Specifically, with Biphasic calcium sulfate/hydroxyapatite (BCS/HA): BCS-CaSO$_4$·1/2 H$_2$O+CaSO$_4$·2H$_2$O and HA-Ca$_{10}$(PO$_4$)$_6$(OH)$_2$ and liquid-NaCl 0.9%.

The selected studies were assessed following the SORT criteria [27].

3. Results

3.1. Selection of Studies

The initial search yielded 122 articles. After applying the inclusion criteria and eliminating duplicate entries, the selected studies were 37. After reading the abstracts, 17 studies were selected and finally, after the full reading of the articles, only 7 fulfilled the criteria (Figure 1). The data obtained is summarized in Table 1.

3.2. Study Design

Table (c) was created to extract data from the selected articles [28–34]. The characteristics of the studies, their objectives, and the results and conclusions obtained were assessed separately.

Three randomized controlled clinical trials (RCT) [28,30,31], three controlled clinical trials [29,33,34], and one case series [32] were included. All clinical trials had a control group comparable to the study group, and three of them used the contralateral side as the control group [28,29,31].

According to the SORT criteria [27], we can state that all RCT [28,30,31] are level 1, and the controlled clinical trials [29,33,34] can be marked as level 2, and finally the case series [32] can be staged as a level 3.

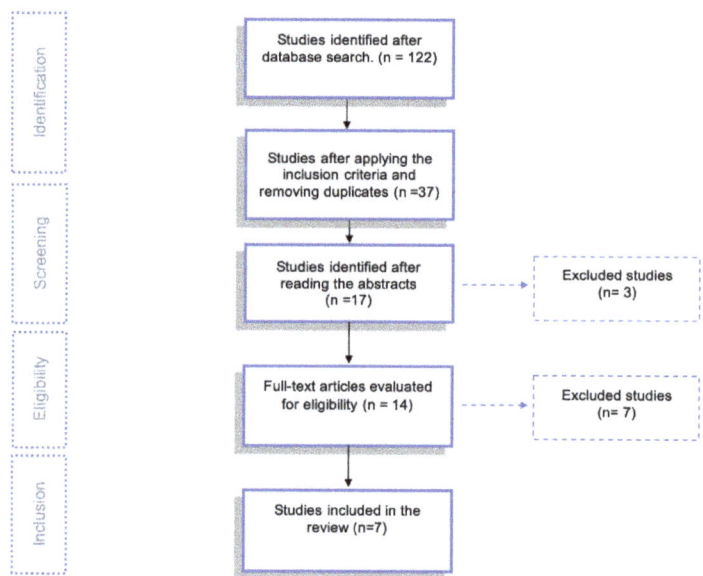

Figure 1. PRISMA flowchart.

3.3. Characteristics of the Participants

A total of 237 patients, with a mean age of 53.95 years, were included in the studies. Only three studies [30,31,33] specify the number of participants of each gender. All the articles except one [28] collected samples from a number equal to or greater than 25 participants, with 60 participants being the maximum [33].

3.4. Characteristics and Results of the Studies

In the selected studies, the applications and efficacy of the use of calcium sulfate in oral surgery were assessed. Two articles evaluated its effectiveness in the treatment of periodontal defects [28,29], three studies evaluated its use as a graft material in alveolar preservation [30,32], and one studied its application in the regeneration of maxillary bone defects after the surgical removal of radicular cysts [33] and another in sinus lifts [34].

Only two authors evaluated the efficacy of calcium sulfate in the guided bone regeneration of periodontal defects. First of all, Pandit et al. [29] obtained a decrease in probing depth of 2.67–4 mm, an increase in the clinical attachment of 1.6–2.47 mm, and a reduction in the periodontal defect of about 2 mm, without observing statistically significant differences between the groups. Secondly, Mandlik et al. [29] obtained a decrease in the probing depth and a gain in the clinical attachment level of about 5 mm in both groups without presenting statistically significant differences.

Of the three studies [30–32] that evaluated the use of calcium sulfate in alveolar preservation procedures, Horowitz et al. [32] reported that bone volume and density were maintained after extractions and after 4 months; Matchei et al. [30] and Mayer et al. [31] instead reported a slight bone loss in height of 0.65 mm [30] and 0.3 mm [31] and width of 0.5 mm [30] and 0.03 mm [31], respectively.

All of the studies performed a histopathological analysis. Matchei et al. [30] reported new bone formation in 44.4% and 16.51% of remnant calcium sulfate. Similar results were found in Mayer et al. [31], who observed that the composition of the new bone consists of 47.7% bone, 36.3% connective tissue, and 16% remaining graft material, and finally Horowitz et al. [32] reported that after 4 months the calcium sulfate graft was reabsorbed completely.

Table 1. Summary of the articles included. RCT: Randomized controlled clinical trial, CT: Controlled clinical trial, CS: Calcium sulfate, NG: Nanogen, DG: Dentogen, BG: BoneGen, BDX: Bovine Xenograft, BCS/HA: Calcium sulfate with hydroxyapatite.

Author/Year Type of Study	Sample Size (n) Gender M/F Age	Type of Study	Results	Conclusions
Pandit et al. [28] 2021 RCT	n: 16 20–64 years old Splitmouth Nanogen n: 15, Dentogen n: 15, BoneGen n: 15	To evaluate the efficacy of calcium sulfate in the treatment of periodontal defects. Comparison of three materials Nanogen (NG), Dentogen (DG), and BoneGen (BG).	At 6 months Probing level reduction: NG 3.33 mm, DG 2.67 mm y BG 4 mm. Clinical insertion gain: NG 1.6 mm, DG 2.20 mm y BG 2.47 mm. Reduction of the periodontal defect: NG 2 mm, DG 2.07 mm, BG 2.07 mm. No statistically significant differences between groups.	Calcium sulfate is an effective material in the treatment of periodontal defects.
Mandlik et al. [29] 2012 CT	n: 25 30–50 years old Splitmouth Group A n: 25, Group B n: 25	To compare the efficacy of phosphosilicate (Group A) and calcium sulfate (Group B) in the treatment of periodontal defects.	At 9 months Probing level: Group A $7.52 \pm 1.074 \rightarrow 2.20 \pm 0.040$ mm Group B $7.20 \pm 1.069 \rightarrow 2.14 \pm 0.351$ mm Clinical insertion level: Group A $7.52 \pm 1.0359 \rightarrow 2.48 \pm 0.614$ mm Group B $7.20 \pm 1.069 \rightarrow 2.32 \pm 0.471$ Bone gain: Group A 58.93%/Group B 48.56% No statistically significant differences between groups.	No significant differences were observed between the two materials in terms of the efficacy of treating periodontal defects.
Machtei et al. [30] 2018 RCT	n: 11 7M/4F 45–80 = 64 years old	To compare the dimensional changes and bone quality of calcium sulfate (BCS/HA) and bovine xenograft (BDX) in socket preservation cases.	At 4 months Bone height loss: BDX 0.25 mm, BCS/HA 0.65 mm, Control 1.7 mm Bone width loss at −3 mm: BDX 1.56 ± 0.4 mm, BCS/HA 0.5 ± 0.4 mm Control 2.96 ± 0.3 mm New bone formation: BDX 21.5%, BCS/HA 44.4% y Control 81.5%. Remaining graft material: BDX 44.18%, BCS/HA 16.51%.	Calcium sulfate can be used as the material of choice for socket preservation with similar and sometimes even better results than bovine xenograft.
Mayer et al. [31] 2016 RCT	n: 36 13M/23F Splitmouth CS n: 14, Control n: 15	To evaluate the efficacy of calcium sulfate in cases of socket preservation.	At 4 months Bone height loss: CS 0.3 ± 2.01, Control 0.1 ± 2.03 Bone width loss at −3 mm: CS 0.03 ± 2.32 mm, Control 2.28 ± 2.36 mm Histopathological analysis: CS 47.7% bone, 36.3% connective tissue graft y 16% remaining graft material Control 52.6% bone y 46.7% connective tissue graft	Calcium sulfate is an effective material in socket preservation cases, providing better results than natural healing.
Horowitz et al. [32] 2012 Case series	n: 40	To evaluate the efficacy of calcium sulfate in cases of socket preservation.	At 4 months Bone volume and density were maintained. Calcium sulfate is completely reabsorbed, giving rise to new bone.	Calcium sulfate is an effective material in cases of socket preservation before implant placement.

Table 1. Cont.

Author/Year Type of Study	Sample Size (n) Gender M/F Age	Type of Study	Results	Conclusions
Dudek et al. [33] 2020 CT	CS n: 30 14M/16F 28–68 = 55.6 years old Xenograft n: 30 14M/16F 27–65 = 61.1 years old	To evaluate the efficacy of calcium sulfate in the regeneration of maxillary bone defects after surgical removal of radicular cysts compared to the use of xenografts.	Calcium sulfate achieves faster bone remodeling than bovine xenograft. Virtually complete reabsorption of calcium sulfate and replacement by new bone at 3 months.	The use of calcium sulfate proved to be a simple, inexpensive, and effective reconstructive treatment of bone defects after the enucleation of odontogenic cysts.
Laino et al. [34] 2015 CT	n: 27 49–75 = 59 years old	To evaluate the efficacy of calcium sulfate in lateral window sinus lifts.	At 6 months Mean bone height before surgery: 4.04 ± 1.48 Mean bone height in regenerated sites: 12.25 ± 3.20 mm Mean bone height gained: 8.21 ± 1.73 mm	The use of calcium sulfate in lateral window sinus lifts is an effective procedure.

Dudek et al. [33] evaluated the efficacy of calcium sulfate in the regeneration of maxillary bone defects after the surgical removal of radicular cysts compared to the use of xenografts and observed that calcium sulfate achieves slightly faster bone remodeling and has almost complete resorption and a new bone replacement at 3 months.

The use of calcium sulfate as a graft material in lateral membrane sinus lifts was evaluated by Laino et al. [34], who obtained a mean bone height gain of 8.21 ± 1.73 mm after 6 months.

4. Clinical Cases

After reviewing the topic, six clinical cases used Bond Apatite® as bone graft material in different procedures. The characteristics of the patients and surgeries are summarized in Table 2.

Table 2. Description of the cases. I.M.: Intraoperative management; I.C.: Intraoperative complications; G: Good; M: Moderate.

Patient Gender Age	Medical History of Interest [Toxic Habits] Type of Surgery	Closure by First Intention [Collagen Sponge]	I.M.	I.C.	Healing	Early Postoperative Complications	Late Postoperative Complications
1 F 63	NO [Tobacco: 2 cig/day] Horizontal Guided Bone Regeneration	Yes [No]	G	No	G	No	No
2 M 52	NO [-] Alveolar ridge preservation	No [Yes]	G	No	M	Graft loss and self-limited alveolitis	No
3 M 61	NO [-] Alveolar ridge preservation	Yes [No]	G	No	G	No	No osseointegration of the implant, replacement in 3 months, without problems and with good stability
4 F 46	NO [-] Alveolar ridge preservation	No [Yes]	G	No	M	Graft loss and self-limited alveolitis	No
5 M 64	NO [-] Sinus lift with lateral window	Yes [No]	G	No	G	No	No
6 M 46	NO [-] Sinus lift with lateral window	Yes [No]	G	No	G	No	No

Without exception, informed consent was obtained from all subjects involved in the study.

In all cases, both after the extractions and after the placement of the implants, post-surgical recommendations were provided and explained, as well as Amoxicillin 750 mg every 8 h × 7 days, Dexketoprofen 25 mg every 8 h × 3–4 days alternated with Paracetamol 1g every 8 h if there was pain, in addition to rinses with Chlorhexidine 0.12% (Bexident® Post topical gel, Isdin, Barcelona Spain) every 8 h × 7 days beginning 24 h after surgery.

Periodic follow-ups were carried out after a week, after the first month, and three months after the intervention with their corresponding X-ray. In all cases except one (Patient No. 1), after 4 months and before implant placement, a biopsy of the regenerated area was performed using a histopathological study (Trefina Komet, 032, Barcelona Spain, 032, diameter 3, 2 external, and 2.6 mm internal).

4.1. Patient No. 1

A 63-year-old woman with no known allergies or medical history of interest, a smoker of two cigarettes a day, came to the clinic to rehabilitate an edentulous area at levels 45 and 47. She presented with 46 with a metal-ceramic crown and cantilever towards the mesial (Figure 2A). It was decided to cut the cantilever, keep the crown at 46 temporarily, place implants at 45 and 47 and subsequently rehabilitate with three individual metal-ceramic crowns. At the 45 level, there was a horizontal bone defect (Figure 2B), so it was decided to perform a lateral ridge augmentation with Bond Apatite® on the same day as implant placement. Surgery was performed following the manufacturer's protocol, incision, detachment of the mucoperiosteal flap, micro-perforations in the cortex, placement of a Bond Apatite® syringe, compression with dry and sterile gauze, placement of Microdent® Genius 3.5 × 12 mm implants at the level of 45 and 4.5 × 12 mm at the level of 47, following the milling of the commercial house, repositioning the flap and tension suture (Figure 3). The recommendations and postoperative pharmacological guidelines were delivered. No intra- or postoperative complications occurred. The stitches were removed a week after surgery (Figure 4A) and regular monthly check-ups were performed (Figure 4B,C). After three months, a new CBCT was requested to assess the bone gain achieved (Figure 2D). Prosthodontic rehabilitation was carried out 4 months after surgery.

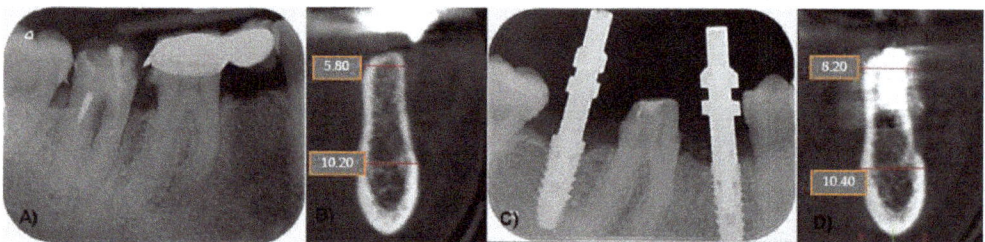

Figure 2. (**A**) Preoperative intraoral periapical radiograph (IOPA); (**B**) Initial CBCT; (**C**) Intraoperative IOPA; (**D**) CBCT after 4 months.

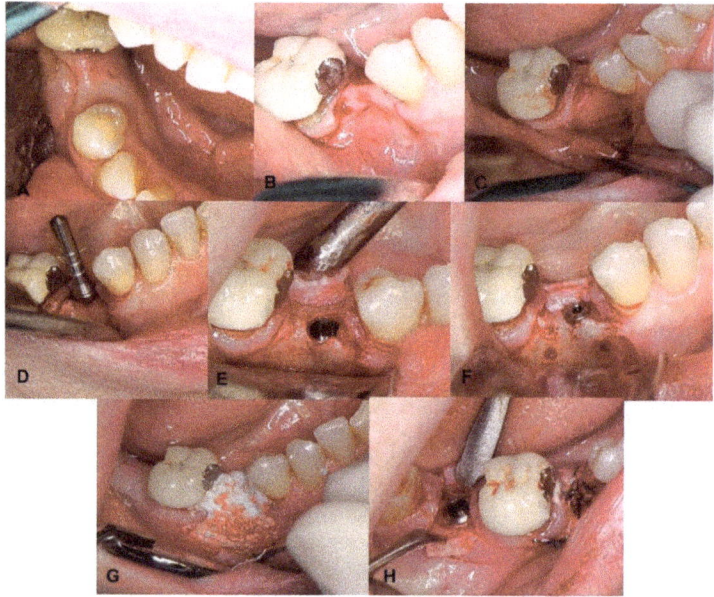

Figure 3. (**A**) Preoperative occlusal view; (**B**) Incision; (**C**) flap detachment; (**D**) Drilling according to protocol, check the position with the pin; (**E**) Implant placement at level 45; (**F**) Micro perforations in the vestibular; (**G**) Placement of Bond Apatite®; (**H**) Tension suture and implant placement in 47.

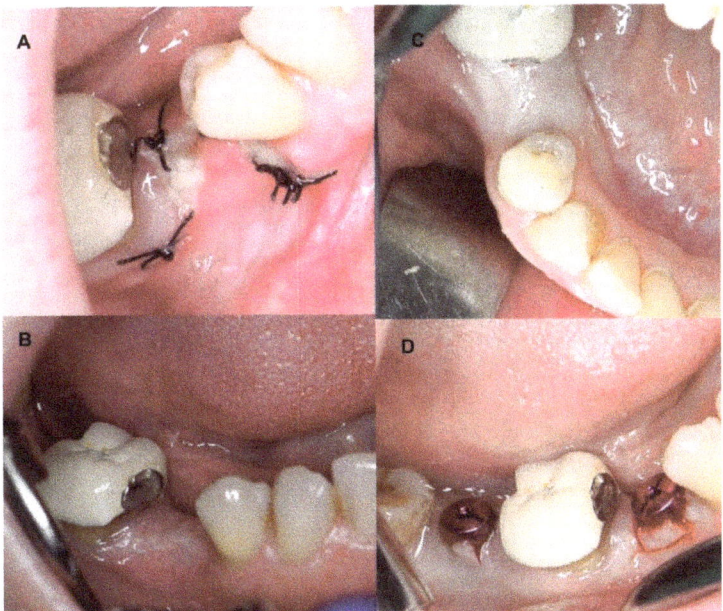

Figure 4. (**A**) Follow-up and removal of the suture after 7 days; (**B**) 1 month follow-up; (**C**) 2 months follow-up; (**D**) 3 months follow-up and healing abutments' placement.

4.2. Patient No. 2

A 52-year-old man with no known allergies or medical or toxicological history of interest came to the clinic to assess the extraction of the 15 root remnant (Figure 5A) and placement of an implant. The case was assessed and, as there was not enough apical bone (Figure 6A), the possibility of placing an implant immediately after extraction was ruled out; it was decided to perform alveolar preservation after extraction and placement of the implant in a second surgical phase. We proceeded to the extraction of 15 and alveolar preservation with Bond Apatite® according to the manufacturer's protocol, extraction, curettage of the alveolus, placement of a Bond Apatite® syringe, compression with dry and sterile gauze, coverage with a collagen sponge and point of cross suture (Figure 7). There were no intraoperative complications. The recommendations and postoperative pharmacological guidelines were delivered. A week later, the patient attended suture removal reporting considerable pain. On examination, alveolitis and loss of graft material were observed, so the medication was changed to Amoxicillin/Clavulanic Acid 875/125 mg every 8 h × 7 days, Dexketoprofen 25mg every 8 h alternated with Metamizole 575 mg every 8 h if there was pain. Periodic monthly follow-ups were carried out (Figure 5B,C) and at 4 months a new CBCT of the area was requested (Figure 6B) for implant planning, where good healing and maintenance of bone volume were observed. On the day of surgery, a trephine biopsy was taken in the regenerated area for histopathological analysis (Figure 8) and a 3.5 × 10 mm Microdent® Genius implant was placed following the milling protocol of the commercial house (Figure 5D). The same pharmacological regimen was prescribed as on the day of the extraction and monthly follow-up visits were scheduled. Currently, he must undergo the second surgical phase and subsequent prosthodontic rehabilitation.

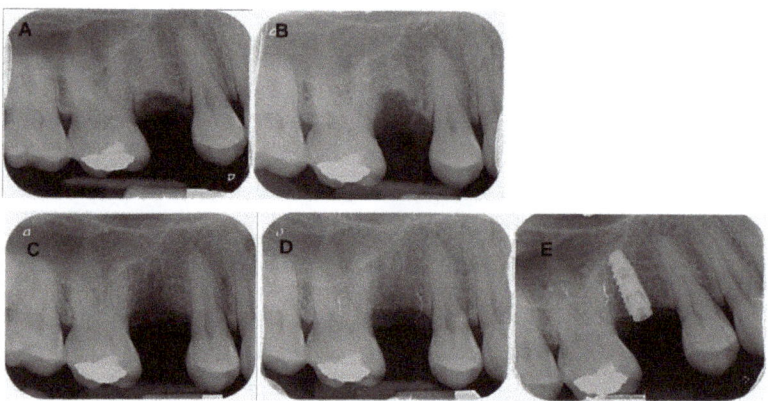

Figure 5. (**A**) Immediate postoperative periapical; (**B**) One week IOPA; (**C**) One month IOPA; (**D**) Two months IOPA; (**E**) IOPA after implant placement.

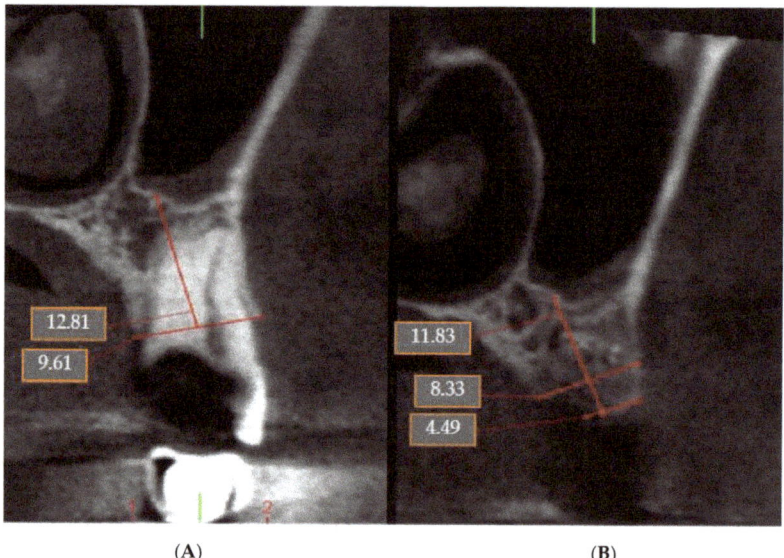

Figure 6. (**A**) Previous CBCT; (**B**) CBCT after 4 months.

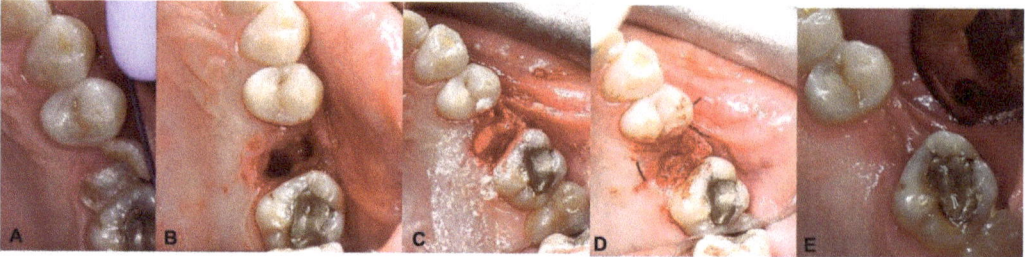

Figure 7. (**A**) Preoperative occlusal view; (**B**) Dental extraction of 25; (**C**) Placement of Bond Apatite®; (**D**) Postoperative occlusal view; (**E**) One-week follow-up.

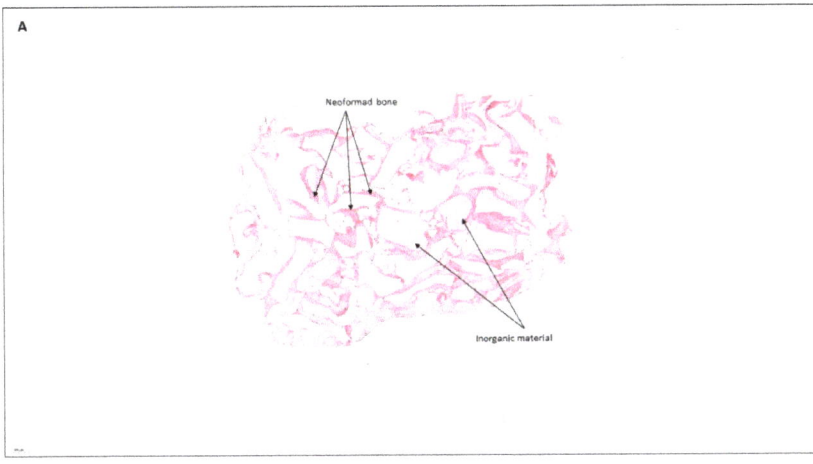

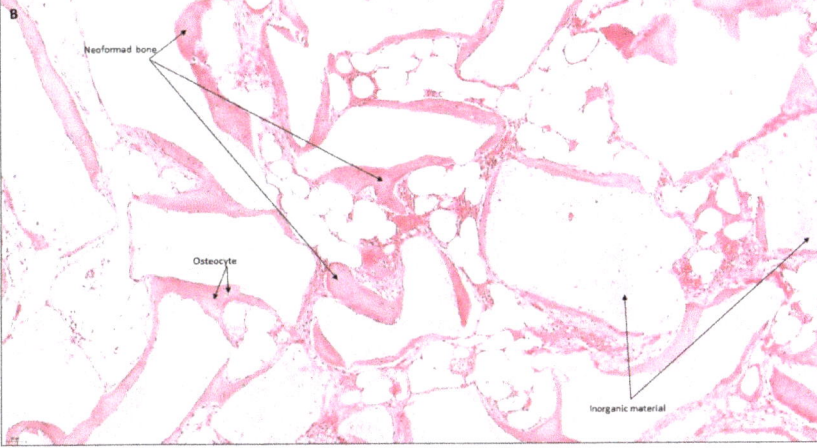

Figure 8. (**A**) Remains of inorganic material with newly formed bone trabeculae in (**A**) at 50× and in (**B**) at 200×. Total bone length of 5.97 mm and newformed bone of 2.98 mm.

4.3. Patient No. 3

A 61-year-old male with no known allergies or relevant medical or toxicological history presented with pain in 24. He had a 24 endodontic treatment, with a filtered metal-ceramic crown in the distal part, non-restorable caries, so extraction was decided (Figure 9A). A CBCT was requested to assess the possibility of immediate implant placement, but the option was ruled out due to the presence of an apical lesion (Figure 10A). It was decided to perform alveolar preservation after extraction and placement of the implant in a second surgical phase. We proceeded to extract 24, profuse curettage of the alveolus, placement of a Bond Apatite® syringe, compression with dry and sterile gauze, and instead of placing a collagen sponge, the manufacturer's protocol was slightly changed since the closure was carried out by primary intention using a vestibular mucoperiosteal flap (Figure 11). There were no intraoperative complications. The recommendations and postoperative pharmacological guidelines were delivered. The stitches were removed a week after surgery and regular monthly check-ups were performed (Figure 9B–E). At 4 months, a new CBCT of the area was requested for implant planning, where good healing and maintenance of bone volume were observed (Figure 10C). On the day of surgery, a trephine biopsy was taken in the regenerated area for histopathological analysis (Figure 12) and a 3.5 × 12 mm

Microdent® Genius implant was placed following the milling protocol of the commercial house (Figure 9F). The same pharmacological regimen was prescribed as on the day of the extraction and monthly follow-up visits were scheduled. Four months after the placement of the implant, the second surgical phase was performed and at the time of removal of the closure plug, the implant was explanted in its entirety, showing the lack of osseointegration of it, a profuse curettage of the area and the implant replacement visit was scheduled after 3 months.

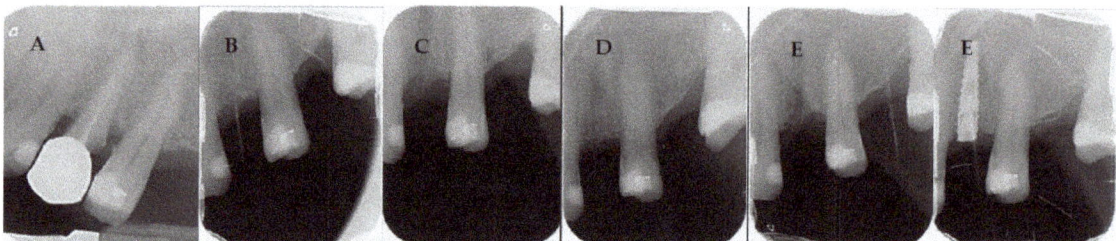

Figure 9. (**A**) Preoperative IOPA; (**B**) Immediate postoperative IOPA; (**C**) One week IOPA; (**D**) One month IOPA; (**E**) Two months IOPA; (**F**) IOPA after implant placement.

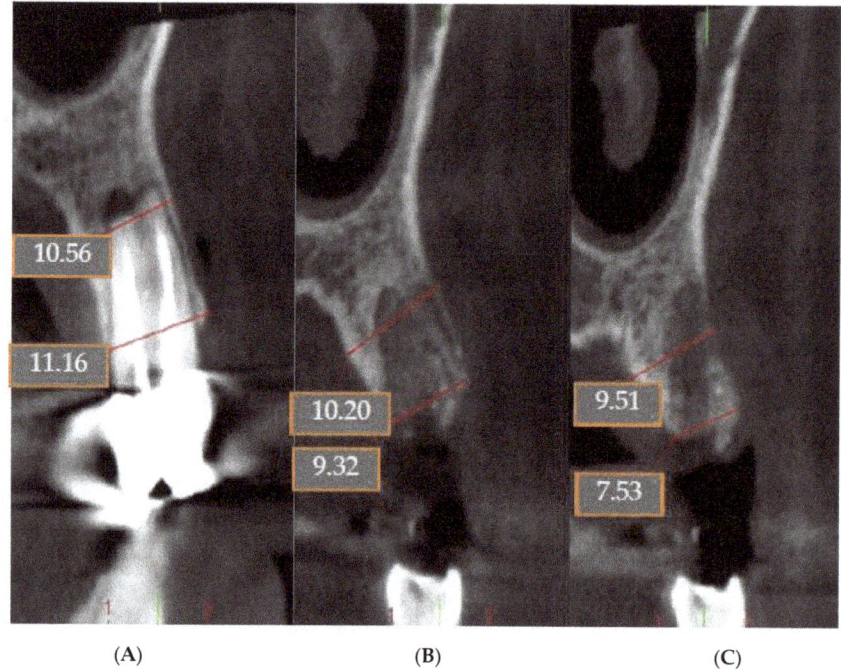

Figure 10. (**A**) Previous CBCT; (**B**) Immediate postoperative CBCT; (**C**) Postoperative CBCT after 4 months.

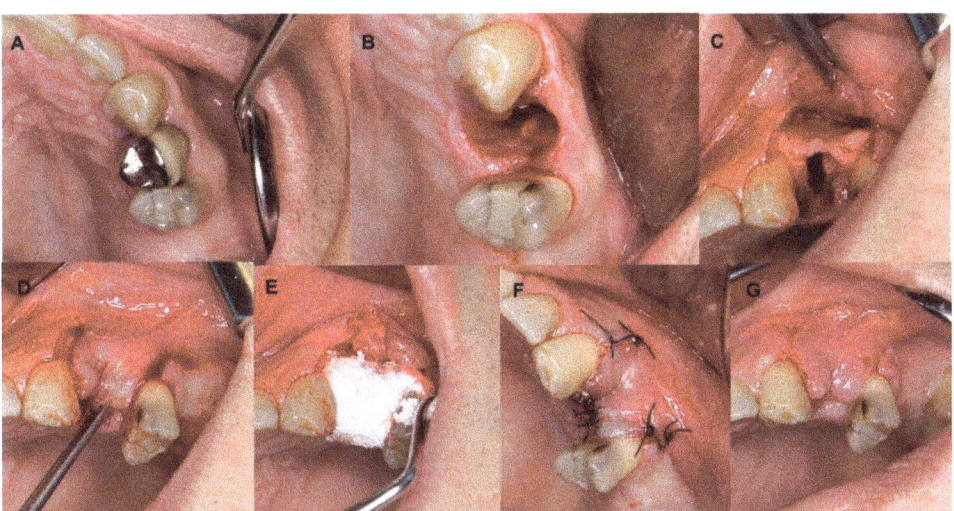

Figure 11. (**A**) Preoperative occlusal view; (**B**) Dental extraction of 24; (**C**) Mucoperiosteal flap; (**D**) Passivity check; (**E**) Placement of Bond Apatite®; (**F**) Closing by the first intention; (**G**) One-week follow-up.

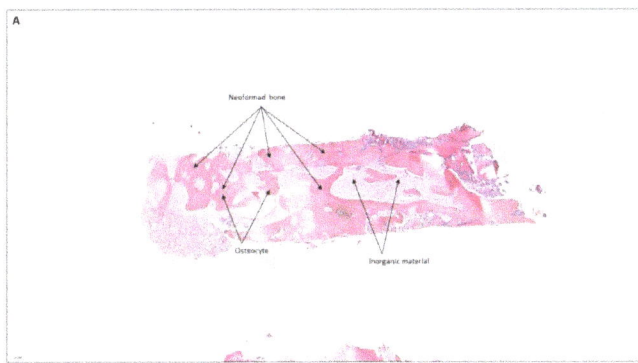

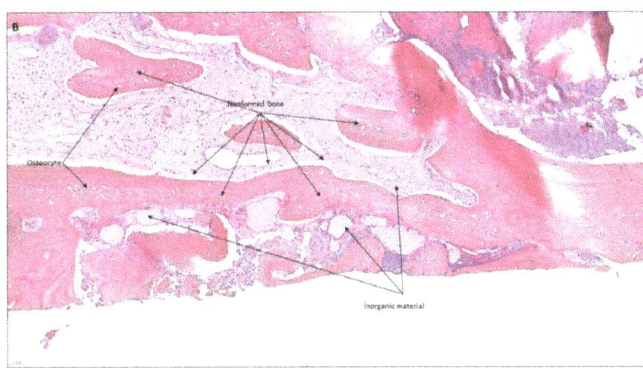

Figure 12. Remains of inorganic material and abundant newformed bone. Some degree of spinal cord fibrosis. (**A**) at 50× and (**B**) at 200×. Total bone length is 4.7 mm and newformed bone is 2.34 mm.

4.4. Patient No.4

A 46-year-old woman with no known allergies or relevant medical or toxicological history came to the clinic due to discomfort in the upper-anterior area. She presented 12, 11, 21, and 22 with metal-ceramic crowns, endodontics, with apical lesions in all of them, and fistulas in the palatal area (Figure 13A). The patient explained that root canal retreatment had already been carried out on these teeth, so conservative treatment was ruled out and it was decided to extract all of them. A CBCT of the area was requested to assess the possible placement of immediate implants, but after observing the apical lesions (Figures 14 and 15), it was decided to place them in a second surgical phase. The 12, 11, 21, and 22 were extracted and an alveolar preservation with Bond Apatite® was performed according to the manufacturer's protocol, extraction, profuse curettage of the alveolus, placement of a Bond Apatite® syringe, compression with dry and sterile gauze, coverage with collagen sponge and cross stitches (Figure 15A–D). There were no intraoperative complications. Pharmacological recommendations and guidelines were delivered. A week later, the patient came to have the suture removed, reporting pain. On examination, alveolitis and loss of graft material were observed (Figure 15E). Amoxicillin/clavulanic acid 875/125 mg every 8 h × 7 days was prescribed. Periodic monthly check-ups were performed (Figure 13B–E) and at 4 months a new CBCT of the area was requested for implant planning, where good healing and maintenance of bone volume were observed (Figure 16). On the day of surgery, a trephine biopsy was taken in the regenerated area for histopathological analysis (Figure 17) and two 4.2 × 12 mm Microdent® Genius implants were placed in positions 12 and 22 following the drilling protocol for the commercial house (Figure 13F). The same pharmacological regimen was prescribed on the day of the extraction and monthly follow-up visits were scheduled. An immediate provisional screw-retained prosthesis was made and placed. Currently, he must undergo the second surgical phase and subsequent definitive prosthodontic rehabilitation.

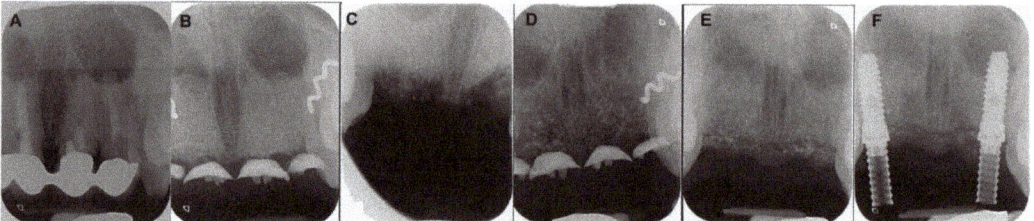

Figure 13. (**A**) Preoperative IOPA; (**B**) Immediate postoperative IOPA; (**C**) One-week IOPA; (**D**) One-month IOPA; (**E**) Two months IOPA; (**F**) IOPA after implant placement.

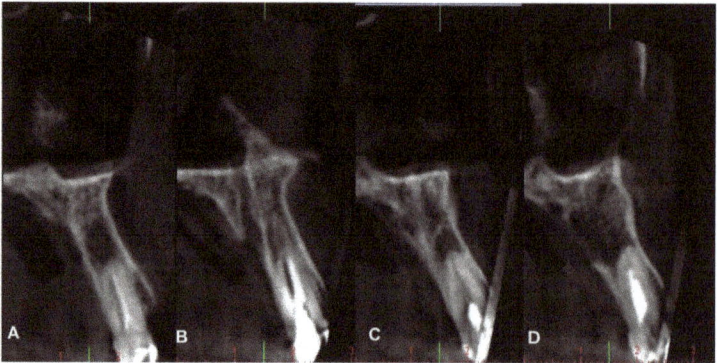

Figure 14. Previous CBCT. (**A**) 12 (**B**) 11 (**C**) 21 (**D**) 22.

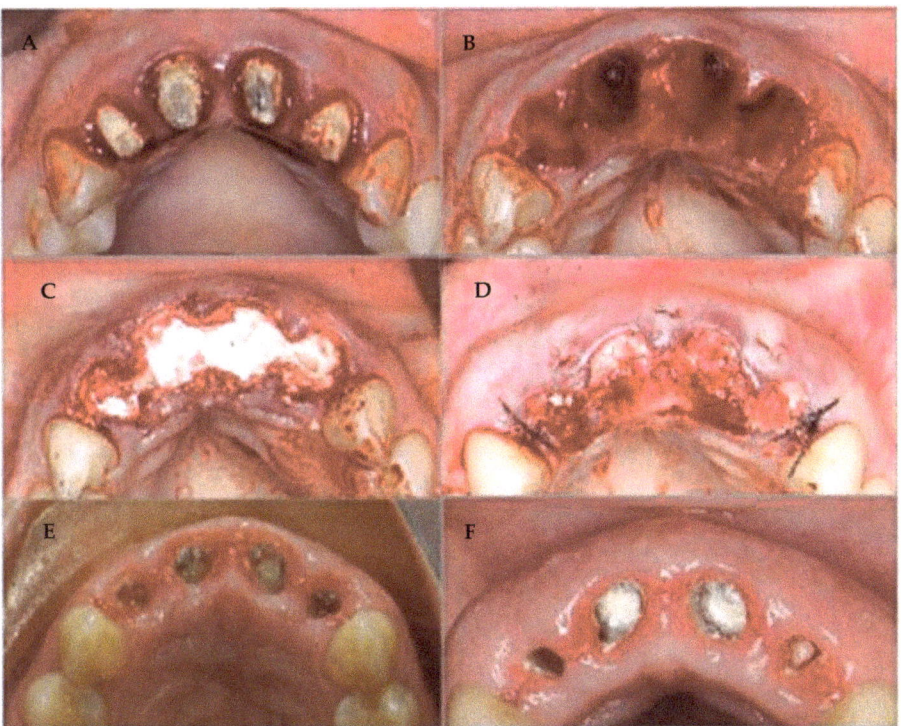

Figure 15. (**A**) Preoperative occlusal view; (**B**) Dental extractions; (**C**) Placement of Bond Apatite®; (**D**) Suture; (**E**) 7 days' follow-up; (**F**) 15 days' follow-up.

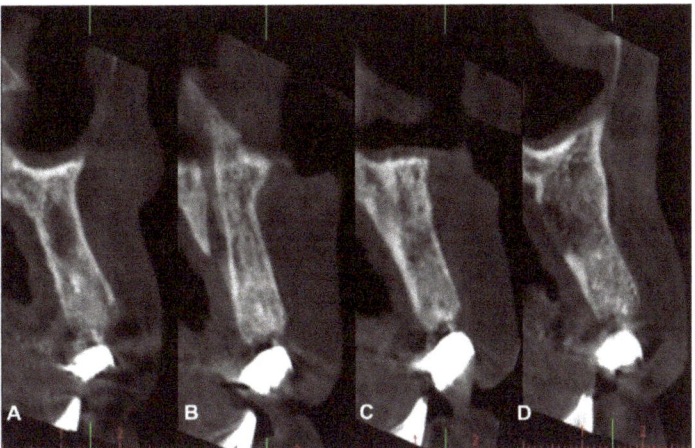

Figure 16. Postoperative CBCT after 4 months. (**A**) 12 (**B**) 11 (**C**) 21 (**D**) 22.

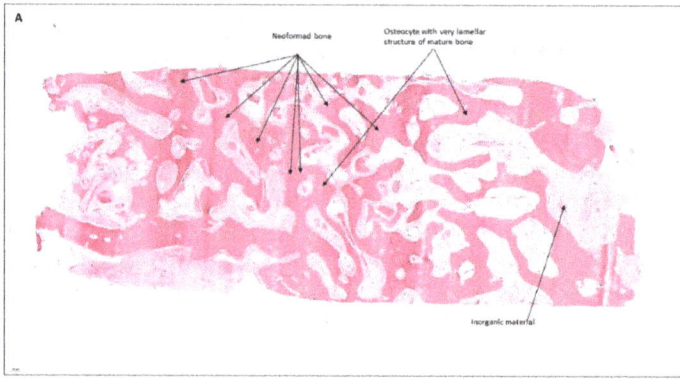
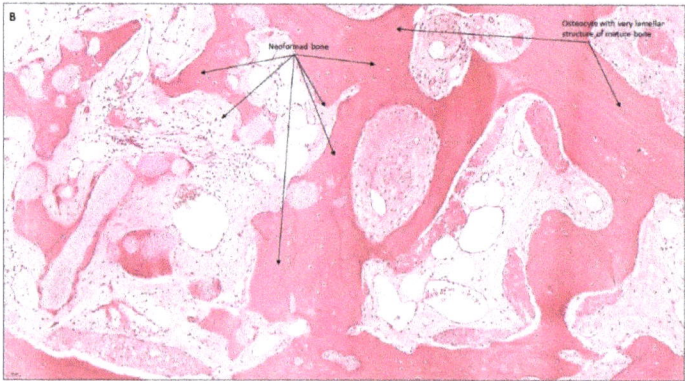

Figure 17. Few remains of inorganic material and abundant newly formed bone. (**A**) at 50× and (**B**) at 200×. Total bone length 6.63 mm, and clearly newformed bone indistinguishable from the rest 3.53 mm.

4.5. Patient No.5

A 64-year-old male with no known allergies or medical or toxicological history of interest came to the clinic to assess rehabilitation of the second edentulous posterior quadrant by placing implants. CBCT was performed (Figure 18A) to assess bone availability in the area. It was observed that it was necessary to perform a sinus lift with a lateral window to have sufficient bone availability for the dental implant placement of 26 (3.6 mm height). It was decided to use Bond Apatite® as the bone graft material. On the day of surgery, the manufacturer's protocol was followed, detachment of the mucoperiosteal flap, preparation of the window and detachment of the sinus membrane, activation of the Bond Apatite® syringe and waiting for 1 min, placement of Bond Apatite® in the mesial area and compression with a periosteotome wrapped in a dry and sterile gauze, placement of Bond Apatite® in the distal and medial area until the cavity is filled, compression with a dry and sterile gauze from the outside of the window, reposition of the flap and suture under tension (Figure 19). Two syringes of Bond Apatite® were used. No intraoperative complications occurred and a CBCT was performed immediately after surgery (Figure 19) where a bone height gain of 12.6 mm was observed. Postoperative recommendations and pharmacological regimens were delivered. Periodic monthly check-ups were performed and at 4 months a new CBCT was requested (Figure 18C) of the area for implant planning, where good healing and bone height gain of 5.6mm were observed, a surprising result since it means that, after 4 months, more than 50% had been lost on the day of surgery.

On the day of implant placement, a trephine biopsy was taken in the regenerated area for histopathological analysis (Figure 20) and a 4.25 × 10 mm Microdent® Genius implant was placed at 26 following the drilling protocol of the commercial house. The same pharmacological regimen was prescribed as on the day of the sinus lift, and monthly follow-up visits were scheduled. Three months after the placement of the implant, the second surgical phase was carried out, and prosthodontic rehabilitation is currently being carried out.

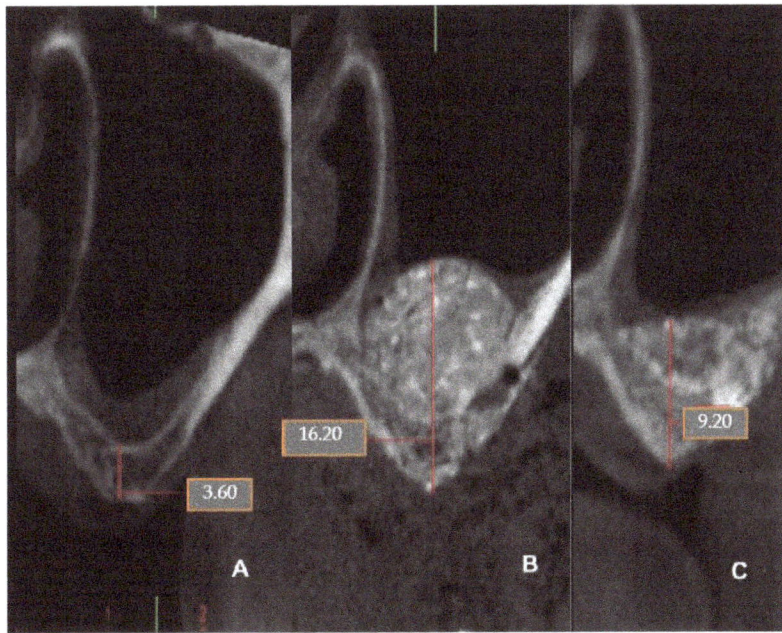

Figure 18. (**A**) Preoperative CBCT; (**B**) Immediate postoperative CBCT; (**C**) Postoperative CBCT after 4 months.

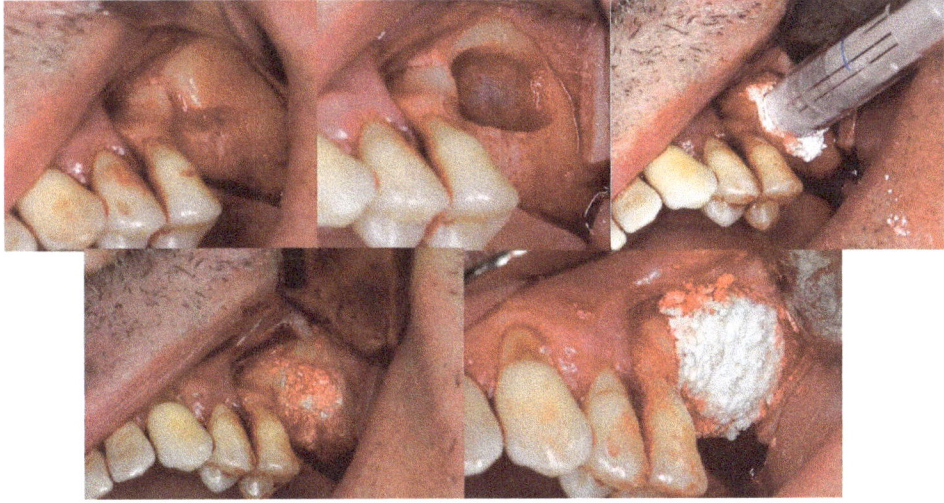

Figure 19. Intraoperative photographs.

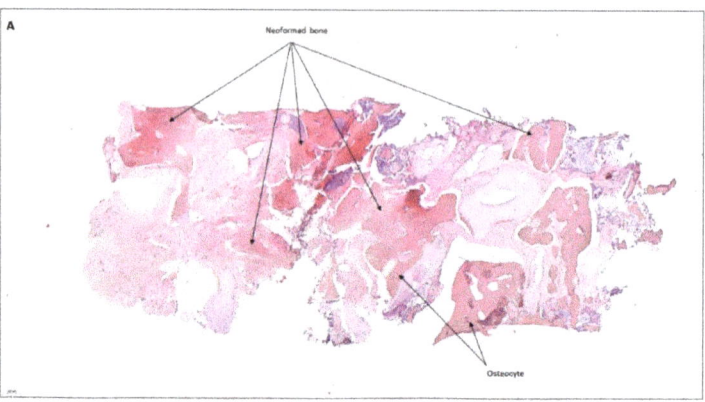

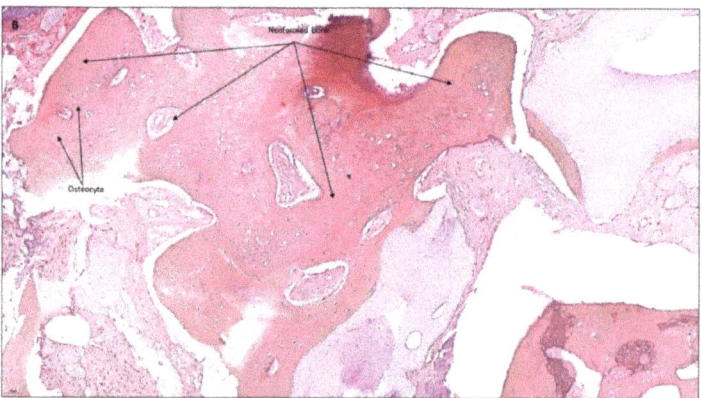

Figure 20. Abundant newly formed bone in (**A**) at 50× and in (**B**) at 200×. Total bone length is 7.2 mm and newly formed bone is 5.4 mm.

4.6. Patient No.6

A 46-year-old man with no known allergies or relevant medical or toxicological history came to the clinic to assess rehabilitation of the edentulous second posterior quadrant by placing implants. CBCT was performed (Figure 21A) to assess bone availability in the area. It was observed that it is necessary to perform a sinus lift with a lateral window to have sufficient bone availability for implant placement since there was 6 mm in the 2.4 mm area and 2.8 mm in the 26 area. It was decided to use Bond Apatite® as the bone graft material. On the day of surgery, the manufacturer's protocol was followed, detachment of the mucoperiosteal flap, preparation of the window and detachment of the sinus membrane, activation of the Bond Apatite® syringe and waiting for 1 min, placement of Bond Apatite® in the mesial area and compression with a periosteotome wrapped in a dry and sterile gauze, placement of Bond Apatite® in the distal and medial area until the cavity is filled, compression with a dry and sterile gauze from the outside of the window, reposition of the flap and suture under tension. Two syringes of Bond Apatite® were used (Figure 22). No intraoperative complications occurred and a CBCT was performed immediately after surgery (Figure 21B) where a bone height gain of 6mm was observed in the mesial area and 9mm in the most distal part. Postoperative recommendations and pharmacological regimens were delivered. Periodic monthly check-ups were performed and at 4 months a new CBCT of the area was requested (Figure 21C) for implant planning, where good healing and bone height gain of 6mm in the mesial area and 9mm in the distal area were observed.

Currently, the patient must undergo implant placement surgery and subsequently a second surgical phase and definitive prosthodontic rehabilitation. The results of the bone biopsy are shown in Figure 23.

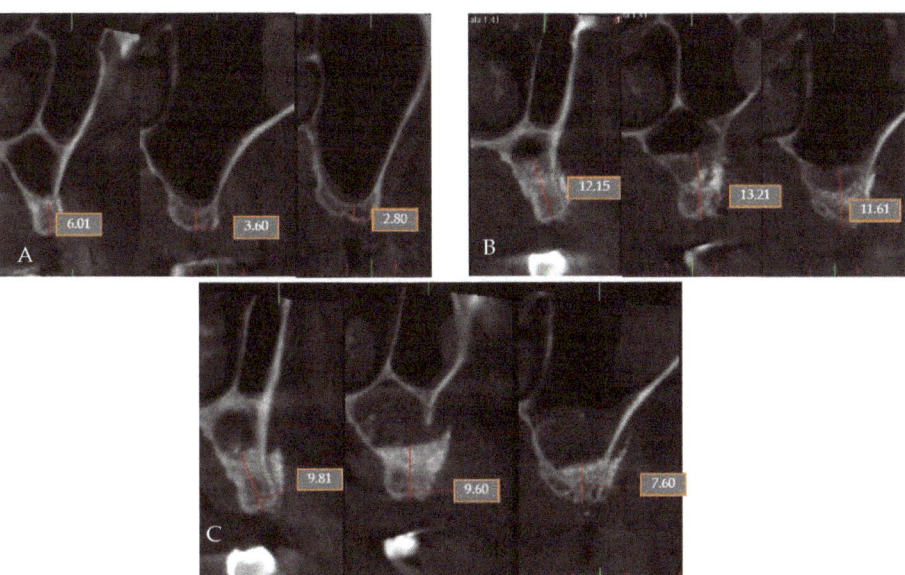

Figure 21. (**A**) Preoperative CBCT at level 24, 25, and 26; (**B**) Immediate postoperative CBCT at level 24, 25, and 26; (**C**) Postoperative CBCT after 4 months at level 24, 25, and 26.

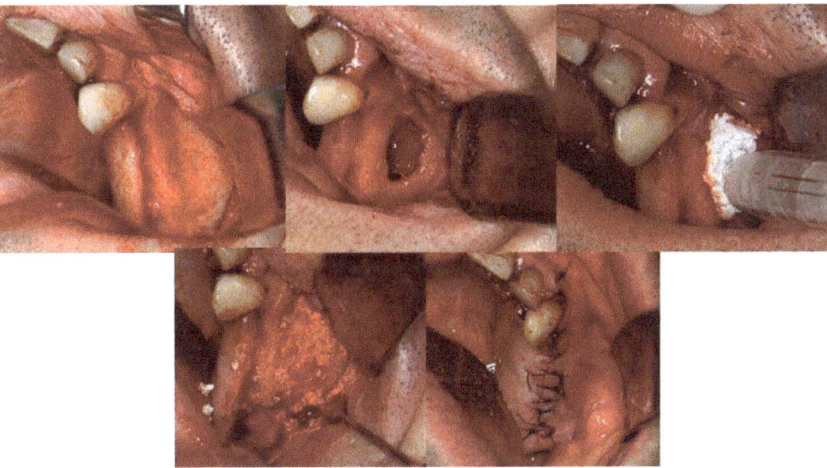

Figure 22. Intraoperative photographs.

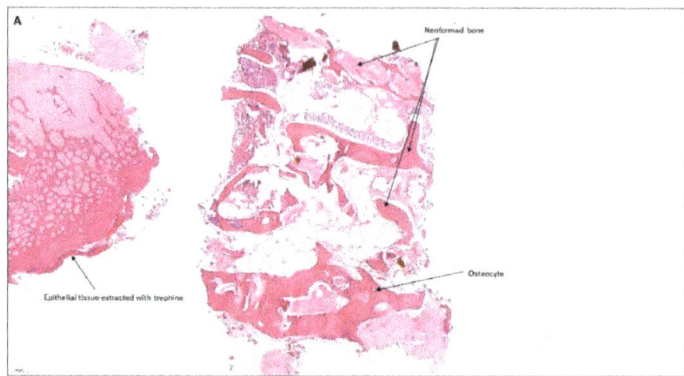
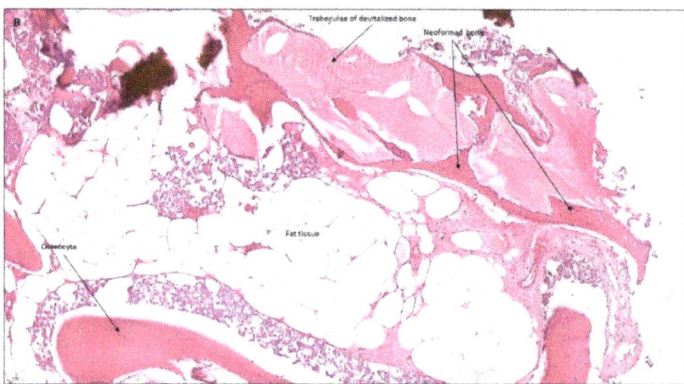
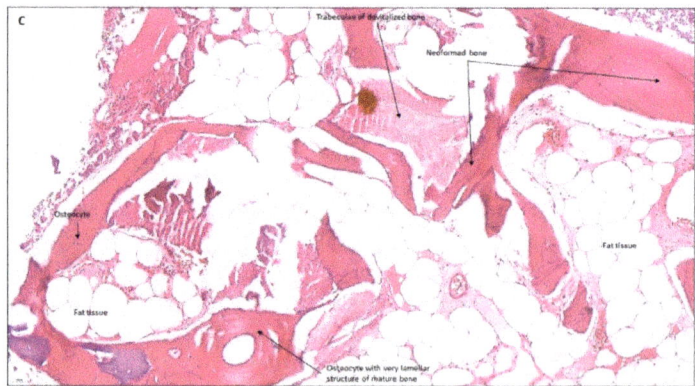

Figure 23. Abundant newly formed bone and some trabeculae of devitalized bone in (**A**) at 50× and in (**B**,**C**) at 200×. Total bone length of 3.56 and newly formed bone of 3.01 mm.

5. Discussion

In this review, the number of articles included was limited due to the limited bibliography on the subject; in addition, most of the included studies had a low level of evidence and had small samples. There was a high level of heterogeneity concerning study design, applications of calcium sulfate, and parameters studied. Due to this lack of homogeneity that complicated the interpretation and summary of the results, it was not possible to compare and analyze the data quantitatively.

Maintaining the volume of the bone crest is important if the placement of implants in the area is subsequently planned, which is why alveolar preservation procedures require graft materials with specific characteristics [5,6].

It is important to take into account the speed and rate of resorption of the graft material, as this influences its osteoconductive capacity. Osteoconduction requires that the bone graft substitute have a rate of resorption similar to the rate of new bone formation. If the rate of resorption is faster than the rate of bone growth, the new bone will not have a scaffold to grow on. Conversely, if the graft material resorbs too slowly, it can remain in the bone defect and block new bone ingrowth [35]. In the case of calcium sulfate, it can be concluded that its resorption rate is favorable for the creation of new bone and for the maintenance of bone volume. The studies included in the review observed a 16% [30,31] residual graft after 4 months. Mahesh et al. [36] quantified its presence between 4.3% and 11.5% after 6 months and other studies [37] stated that, 12 months after the placement of calcium sulfate, it is reabsorbed in 99% and is replaced in 85% by new bone. In this regard, the works carried out by Ricci et al. [38] and, among others, Kadhim et al. [39] are very interesting. They determined that CS acts as a bioactive material when placed in a bone environment. By examining the CS during early periods, with histology, BEI, and XRM, Ricci et al. [38] observed that the CS material did not simply dissolve. As it dissolved and receded, it left behind a consistent latticework of a hydroxyapatite-like calcium phosphate mineral that was stable: in the short term, acted as an osteoconductive trellis for new bone formation, became incorporated in the new bone, and was then remodeled as the bone matured. On the other hand, the main difference between the bioactive glass (BG) and Bond Apatite (biphasic calcium sulfate/hydroxyapatite, BCS/HA) is that the latter (after activation) is injected into the site and can be molded according to the needs of the clinician. It does not require membrane coverage during the augmentation procedure [38].

The alveolar preservation cases that we performed (Case No. 2, Case No. 3, and Case No. 4) using Bond Apatite® as bone regeneration material, obtained good results in terms of maintaining bone volume. It should be noted that, in the cases where the protocol was followed, and closure was not performed by the first intention, alveolitis and partial loss of part of the material were observed after a week (Case No. 2 and Case No. 4); no difficulty was presented for the subsequent insertion of the implants.

Bone grafts continue to be one of the most widely used therapeutic strategies for the correction of periodontal bone defects. Both Trombelli et al. [40] and Reynolds et al. [41] in their systematic reviews summarized that bone substitutes were significantly more effective than open flap debridement in improving attachment levels and reducing probing depth. Both Pandit et al. [28] and Mandlik et al. [29] agree that calcium sulfate is an effective material in the treatment of periodontal defects since it is biocompatible, bioabsorbable, osteoconductive, versatile, and easy to apply. The good results of this material encourage testing its use in peri-implant treatments as it would provide a quick, comfortable, and economical solution for the follow-up of peri-implantitis. Guarnini et al. [42] propose a treatment combining the surface treatment of the implant with powdered abrasives and the use of calcium sulfate as grafting material, obtaining good results.

Laino et al. [33] studied the use of calcium sulfate as a graft in sinus lifts with a lateral window, obtaining good results, including a gain in bone height of more than 8mm, and these results coincide with those of other studies, such as that of Guarnieri et al. [42] who obtained a mean increase in bone height of 8 mm after 6 months and 2 years or that of Kher et al. [43], who reported a slightly greater gain of 10.31 mm. In our series of cases at 4 months, a bone gain of 6 mm and 9 mm was obtained depending on the area in the first case (Case No. 5) and 5.6 mm in the second case (Case No. 6). In the second case, the loss of more than 50% of bone height achieved was surprising when comparing the day of surgery with the follow-up after 4 months.

It is important to consider the size of the defect since it has been established that the width at the base of the defect facilitates space provision and influences bone repair through GBR [44]. Evidently, in tiny faults, the demand for augmentation and consequently the projected gain is slightly smaller than in bigger defects [45]. Large defect augmentation appears to be more difficult and technique-dependent.

Other factors that should be taken into consideration are the location of the defect, since the anterior and posterior mandible and maxilla segments have differing bone properties [46], and the loading timing, since according to the literature, GBR around immediate dental implant placement can improve hard tissue response during the healing period [47].

6. Conclusions

Calcium sulfate as a graft material in oral surgery has proven to be an effective, predictable, practical, economical, and easy-to-handle material in different areas of implant surgery.

Currently, the available literature on the use of calcium sulfate as a graft material in implant surgery is scarce, and what is available provides low-quality evidence. That is why more research studies on the subject are necessary to allow more comparisons and meaningful conclusions.

After using Bond Apatite® in our case series, we can conclude that it is a useful and easy-to-handle material in implantology practice, but more controlled studies should be carried out in this regard to assess its long-term efficacy, especially in horizontal and/or vertical regeneration.

Author Contributions: Conceptualization, J.L.-L. and A.M.-R.; methodology, A.T.-M.; software, B.G.-N.; validation, J.L.-L., A.T.-M. and B.G.-N.; formal analysis, A.A; investigation, A.A; resources, R.Z.-L.G.; data curation, R.Z.-L.G.; writing—original draft preparation, A.A.; writing—review and editing, A.T.-M.; visualization, J.L.-L.; supervision, J.L.-L.; project administration, A.M.-R.; funding acquisition, R.Z.-L.G. All authors have read and agreed to the published version of the manuscript.

Funding: There was no additional funding for this study.

Institutional Review Board Statement: The study was conducted in accordance with the Declaration of Helsinki, the approval by the Institutional Review Board was not required since the data are properly anonymized and informed consent was obtained at the time of original data collection.

Informed Consent Statement: Informed consent was obtained from all subjects involved in the study.

Data Availability Statement: Not applicable.

Acknowledgments: August Vidal Bel of the Pathological Anatomy Service of the Bellvitge University Hospital (HUB).

Conflicts of Interest: The authors declare no conflict of interest.

References

1. Pietrokovski, J.; Massler, M. Alveolar ridge resorption following tooth extraction. *J. Prosthet. Dent.* **1967**, *17*, 21–27. [CrossRef]
2. Youngson, C. Summary of: The influence of specialty training, experience, discussion and reflection on decision making in modern restorative treatment planning. *Br. Dent. J.* **2011**, *210*, 164–165. [CrossRef] [PubMed]
3. Irinakis, T. Rationale for socket preservation after extraction of a single-rooted tooth when planning for future implant placement. *J. Can. Dent. Assoc.* **2006**, *72*, 917–922. [PubMed]
4. Tan, W.L.; Wong, T.L.T.; Wong, M.C.M.; Lang, N.P. A systematic review of post-extractional alveolar hard and soft tissue dimensional changes in humans. *Clin. Oral Implants Res.* **2012**, *23* (Suppl. 5), 1–21. [CrossRef] [PubMed]
5. Iasella, J.M.; Greenwell, H.; Miller, R.L.; Hill, M.; Drisko, C.; Bohra, A.A.; Scheetz, J.P. Ridge preservation with freeze-dried bone allograft and a collagen membrane compared to extraction alone for implant site development: A clinical and histologic study in humans. *J. Periodontol.* **2003**, *74*, 990–999. [CrossRef]
6. Turri, A.; Dahlin, C. Comparative maxillary bone-defect healing by calcium-sulphate or deproteinized bovine bone particles and extra cellular matrix membranes in a guided bone regeneration setting: An experimental study in rabbits. *Clin. Oral Implants Res.* **2015**, *26*, 501–506. [CrossRef]
7. Dahlin, C.; Linde, A.; Gottlow, J.; Nyman, S. Healing of Bone Defects by Guided Tissue Regeneration. *Plast. Reconstr. Surg.* **1988**, *81*, 672–676. [CrossRef]

8. Jung, R.E.; Fenner, N.; Hämmerle, C.H.; Zitzmann, N.U. Long-term outcome of implants placed with guided bone regeneration (GBR) using resorbable and non-resorbable membranes after 12–14 years. *Clin. Oral Implants Res.* **2013**, *24*, 1065–1073. [CrossRef]
9. Chau, A.M.T.; Mobbs, R.J. Bone graft substitutes in anterior cervical discectomy and fusion. *Eur. Spine J.* **2009**, *18*, 449–464. [CrossRef]
10. Bohner, M. Resorbable biomaterials as bone graft substitutes. *Mater. Today* **2010**, *13*, 24–30. [CrossRef]
11. Raghoebar, G.M.; Louwerse, C.; Kalk, W.W.I.; Vissink, A. Morbidity of chin bone harvesting. *Clin. Oral Implants Res.* **2001**, *12*, 503–507. [CrossRef]
12. Younger, E.M.; Chapman, M.W. Morbidity at bone graft donor sites. *J. Orthop. Trauma* **1989**, *3*, 192–195. [CrossRef]
13. Baranes, D.; Kurtzman, G.M. Biphasic Calcium Sulfate as an Alternative Grafting Material in Various Dental Applications. *J. Oral Implant.* **2019**, *45*, 247–255. [CrossRef]
14. Peltier, L.F.; Bickel, E.Y.; Lillo, R.; Thein, M.S. The Use of Plaster of Paris to Fill Defects in Bone. *Ann. Surg.* **1957**, *146*, 61–69. [CrossRef]
15. Thomas, M.V.; Puleo, D.A. Calcium sulfate: Properties and clinical applications. *J. Biomed. Mater. Res. Part B Appl. Biomater.* **2009**, *88*, 597–610. [CrossRef]
16. Walsh, W.R.; Morberg, P.; Yu, Y.; Yang, J.L.; Haggard, W.; Sheath, P.C.; Svehla, M.; Bruce, W.J. Response of a calcium sulfate bone graft substitute in a confined cancellous defect. *Clin. Orthop. Relat. Res.* **2003**, *406*, 228–236. [CrossRef]
17. Crespi, R.; Capparé, P.; Gherlone, E. Magnesium-Enriched Hydroxyapatite Compared to Calcium Sulfate in the Healing of Human Extraction Sockets: Radiographic and Histomorphometric Evaluation at 3 Months. *J. Periodontol.* **2009**, *80*, 210–218. [CrossRef]
18. Gitelis, S.; Piasecki, P.; Turner, T.; Haggard, W.; Charters, J.; Urban, R. Use of a calcium sulfate-based bone graft substitute for benign bone lesions. *Orthopedics* **2001**, *24*, 162–166. [CrossRef]
19. Deliberador, T.M.; Nagata, M.J.; Furlaneto, F.A.; Melo, L.G.; Okamoto, T.; Sundefeld, M.L.; Fucini, S.E. Autogenous Bone Graft with or Without a Calcium Sulfate Barrier in the Treatment of Class II Furcation Defects: A Histologic and Histometric Study in Dogs. *J. Periodontol.* **2006**, *77*, 780–789. [CrossRef]
20. Mayer, Y.; Zigdon-Giladi, H.; Machtei, E.E. Ridge Preservation Using Composite Alloplastic Materials: A Randomized Control Clinical and Histological Study in Humans. *Clin. Implant Dent. Relat. Res.* **2016**, *18*, 1163–1170. [CrossRef]
21. Machtei, E.E.; Rozitsky, D.; Zigdon-Giladi, H.; Levin, L. Bone preservation in dehiscence-type defects using composite biphasic calcium sulfate plus biphasic hydroxyapatite/β-tricalcium phosphate graft: A histomorphometric case series in canine mandible. *Implant Dent.* **2013**, *22*, 590–595. [CrossRef] [PubMed]
22. Brown, M.E.; Zou, Y.; Dziubla, T.D.; Puleo, D.A. Effects of composition and setting environment on mechanical properties of a composite bone filler. *J. Biomed. Mater. Res. A* **2013**, *101*, 973–980. [CrossRef]
23. Wang, L.; Barbieri, D.; Zhou, H.; de Bruijn, J.D.; Bao, C.; Yuan, H. Effect of particle size on osteoinductive potential of microstructured biphasic calcium phosphate ceramic. *J. Biomed. Mater. Res. Part A* **2014**, *103*, 1919–1929. [CrossRef] [PubMed]
24. Yahav, A.; Kurtzman, G.M.; Katzap, M.; Dudek, D.; Baranes, D. Bone Regeneration: Properties and Clinical Applications of Biphasic Calcium Sulfate. *Dent. Clin. N. Am.* **2020**, *64*, 453–472. [CrossRef]
25. Pecora, G.; Andreana, S.; Margarone, J.E., 3rd; Covani, U.; Sottosanti, J.S. Bone regeneration with a calcium sulfate barrier. *Oral Surg. Oral Med. Oral Pathol. Oral Radiol. Endod.* **1997**, *84*, 424–429. [CrossRef]
26. Strocchi, R.; Orsini, G.; Iezzi, G.; Scarano, A.; Rubini, C.; Pecora, G.; Piattelli, A. Bone regeneration with calcium sulfate: Evidence for increased angiogenesis in rabbits. *J. Oral Implantol.* **2002**, *28*, 273–278. [CrossRef]
27. Ebell, M.H.; Siwek, J.; Weiss, B.D.; Woolf, S.H.; Susman, J.; Ewigman, B.; Bowman, M. Strength of recommendation taxonomy (SORT): A patient-centered approach to grading evidence in the medical literature. *Am. Fam. Physician* **2004**, *69*, 548–556. [CrossRef] [PubMed]
28. Pandit, N.; Sharma, A.; Jain, A.; Bali, D.; Malik, R.; Gugnani, S. The use of nanocrystalline and two other forms of calcium sulfate in the treatment of infrabony defects: A clinical and radiographic study. *J. Indian Soc. Periodontol.* **2015**, *19*, 545–553.
29. Mandlik, V.; Roy, S.; Jha, A. Comparative evaluation of bioglass with calcium sulphate β-hemihydrate for the treatment of intraosseous defects—A clinico-radiological study. *Med. J. Armed Forces India* **2012**, *68*, 42–47. [CrossRef]
30. Machtei, E.E.; Mayer, Y.; Horwitz, J.; Zigdon-Giladi, H. Prospective randomized controlled clinical trial to compare hard tissue changes following socket preservation using alloplasts, xenografts vs no grafting: Clinical and histological findings. *Clin. Implant Dent. Relat. Res.* **2018**, *21*, 14–20. [CrossRef]
31. Lindhe, J.; Araújo, M.G.; Bufler, M.; Liljenberg, B. Biphasic alloplastic graft used to preserve the dimension of the edentulous ridge: An experimental study in the dog. *Clin Oral Implants Res.* **2013**, *24*, 1158–1163. [CrossRef]
32. A Horowitz, R.; Rohrer, M.D.; Prasad, H.S.; Tovar, N.; Mazor, Z. Enhancing extraction socket therapy with a biphasic calcium sulfate. *Compend. Contin. Educ. Dent.* **2012**, *33*, 420–426, 428.
33. Dudek, D.; Reichmann-Warmusz, E.; Kurtzman, G.M.; Mahesh, L. The use of grafting material biphasic calcium sulfate for the treatment of osseous defects resulting from radicular cysts. Clinical study and six-month follow up. *J. Osseointegr.* **2020**, *12*, 716–721. [CrossRef]
34. Laino, L.; Troiano, G.; Giannatempo, G.; Graziani, U.; Ciavarella, D.; Dioguardi, M.; Muzio, L.L.; Lauritano, F.; Cicciù, M. Sinus Lift Augmentation by Using Calcium Sulphate. A Retrospective 12 Months Radiographic Evaluation Over 25 Treated Italian Patients. *Open Dent. J.* **2015**, *9*, 414–419. [CrossRef]

35. Peltier, L.F.; Jones, R.H. Treatment of unicameral bone cysts by curettage and packing with plaster-of-Paris pellets. *J. Bone Jt. Surg. Am.* **1978**, *60*, 820–822. [CrossRef]
36. Mahesh, L.; A Salama, M.; Kurtzman, G.M.; Joachim, F.P.C. Socket grafting with calcium phosphosilicate alloplast putty: A histomorphometric evaluation. *Compend. Contin. Educ. Dent.* **2012**, *33*, e109–e115.
37. Kelly, C.M.; Wilkins, R.M.; Gitelis, S.; Hartjen, C.; Watson, J.T.; Kim, P.T. The use of a surgical grade calcium sulfate as a bone graft substitute: Results of a multicenter trial. *Clin. Orthop. Relat. Res.* **2001**, *382*, 42–50. [CrossRef]
38. Trombelli, L.; Heitz-Mayfield, L.J.; Needleman, I.; Moles, D.; Scabbia, A. A systematic review of graft materials and biological agents for periodontal intraosseous defects. *J. Clin. Periodontol.* **2002**, *29* (Suppl. 3), 117–135. [CrossRef]
39. Ricci, J.; Alexander, H.; Nadkarni, P.; Hawkins, M.; Turner, J.; Rosenblum, S.; Brezenoff, L.; Deleonardis, D.; Pecora, G. Biological mechanisms of calcium sulfate replacement by bone. In *Bone Engineering*; Em2 Inc.: Mississauga, ON, Canada, 2000; pp. 332–344.
40. Kadhim, D.R.; Hamad, T.I.; Fatalla, A.A. Use of Eggshells as Bone Grafts around Commercially Pure Titanium Implant Screws Coated with Nano Calcium Sulfate. *Int. J. Biomater.* **2022**, *2022*, 8722283. [CrossRef]
41. Reynolds, M.A.; Aichelmann-Reidy, M.E.; Branch-Mays, G.L.; Gunsolley, J.C. The Efficacy of Bone Replacement Grafts in the Treatment of Periodontal Osseous Defects. A Systematic Review. *Ann. Periodontol.* **2003**, *8*, 227–265. [CrossRef]
42. Guarnieri, R.; Grassi, R.; Ripari, M.; Pecora, G. Maxillary sinus augmentation using granular calcium sulfate (surgiplaster sinus): Radiographic and histologic study at 2 years. *Int. J. Periodontics Restor. Dent.* **2006**, *26*, 79–85.
43. Kher, U.; Ioannou, A.L.; Kumar, T.; Siormpas, K.; Mitsias, M.E.; Mazor, Z.; Kotsakis, G.A. A clinical and radiographic case series of implants placed with the simplified minimally invasive antral membrane elevation technique in the poste-rior maxilla. *J. Craniomaxillofac. Surg.* **2014**, *42*, 1942–1947. [CrossRef] [PubMed]
44. Khojasteh, A.; Kheiri, L.; Motamedian, S.R.; Khoshkam, V. Guided bone regeneration for the reconstruction of alveolar bone defects. *Ann. Maxillofac. Surg.* **2017**, *7*, 263–277. [CrossRef] [PubMed]
45. Beitlitum, I.; Artzi, Z.; Nemcovsky, C.E. Clinical evaluation of particulate allogeneic with and without autogenous bone grafts and resorbable collagen membranes for bone augmentation of atrophic alveolar ridges. *Clin. Oral Implants Res.* **2010**, *21*, 1242–1250. [CrossRef]
46. Sakka, S.; Coulthard, P. Bone Quality: A Reality for the Process of Osseointegration. *Implant Dent.* **2009**, *18*, 480–485. [CrossRef]
47. Kinaia, B.M.; Shah, M.; Neely, A.L.; Goodis, H.E. Crestal Bone Level Changes Around Immediately Placed Implants: A Systematic Review and Meta-Analyses With at Least 12 Months' Follow-Up After Functional Loading. *J. Periodontol.* **2014**, *85*, 1537–1548. [CrossRef]

MDPI
St. Alban-Anlage 66
4052 Basel
Switzerland
Tel. +41 61 683 77 34
Fax +41 61 302 89 18
www.mdpi.com

Coatings Editorial Office
E-mail: coatings@mdpi.com
www.mdpi.com/journal/coatings

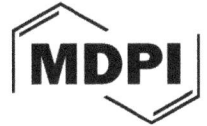

www.ingramcontent.com/pod-product-compliance
Lightning Source LLC
LaVergne TN
LVHW070613100526
838202LV00012B/637